3451|22 43.77

3451|22 43.77

In Their Hands

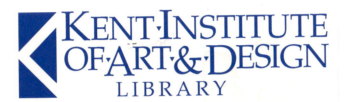
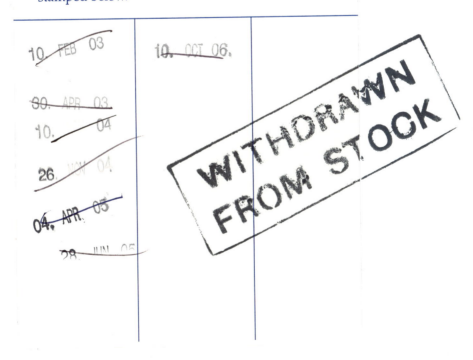
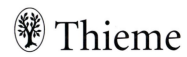 Thieme

IN THEIR HANDS

Photographs by

JAVED SIDDIQI, HBSc, MD, DPHIL(OXON), FRCSC

Program Director and Chief
Department of Neurosurgery
Arrowhead Regional Medical Center
Colton, CA

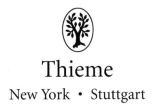

Thieme

New York • Stuttgart

Thieme New York
333 Seventh Avenue
New York, NY 10001

Editor: Felicity Edge
Director, Production and Manufacturing: Anne Vinnicombe
Marketing Director: Phyllis Gold
Sales Manager: Ross Lumpkin
Chief Financial Officer: Peter van Woerden
President: Brian Scanlan
Designer: Marsha Cohen, Parallelogram Graphics
Compositor: Compset, Inc.
Printer: The Maple-Vail Book Manufacturing Company

770.92
779 SID

Library of Congress Cataloging-in-Publication data is available from the publisher

Printed in the United States of America

TNY ISBN 1-58890-083-5
GTV ISBN 3-13-130031-0

CONTENTS

PROLOGUE

This project started over seven years ago after a casual conversation with the late Dr. Charles Drake, one of my neurosurgery mentors in London, Ontario, Canada. I was taking a breather between surgeries, and Dr. Drake was doing the same between chapters of his book on aneurysm surgery. The conversation somehow moved to the concept of "good hands," which for surgeons is a referral to technical prowess; however, early into the conversation it became clear to me that for Drake, the term meant a lot more. With some trepidation I expressed the view that without our hands, the heart and brain would be incomplete. To my pleasant surprise, the great man agreed with me; indeed, he felt that our hands are what give us our humanity, and render us distinct from all other species. Dr. Drake mentioned one trip to Japan where his host had insisted on having his hands molded into bronze statues. In his typical down-to-earth manner, Dr. Drake spoke of how he was given a copy of the final bronze product, a heavy gift he awkwardly "lugged" home with great difficulty. While his humility would not allow him to find anything special in his own hands, he was clearly fascinated with hands of other renowned surgeons. This brief conversation of less than twenty minutes was a watershed in my own fascination with hands. When my idea of black and white photography of neurosurgeons' hands brought a twinkle to Dr. Drake's eyes and a nod of approval, I knew I was onto an idea worth pursuing. Thus, the idea that had been in the back of my mind for some years came to the front, and I started looking for subjects. (Sadly, the photo of Dr. Drake's hands printed in this book was taken in the last few weeks of his life, up until which time he remained an energetic supporter of my photography project.)

A couple of years after the above conversation with Dr. Drake, I found myself in Barcelona, Spain, where I visited the Pablo Picasso museum (formerly the artist's home) and was struck by a painting of a physician seated next to a dying patient. The physician was holding the patient's hand, perhaps simply taking the pulse, but perhaps doing infinitely more. In the whole painting, my eyes repeatedly returned to the two hands. Clearly, in one painting, this artist had managed to capture that which fascinated me about hands, the complexity of the physical and metaphysical nuances of non-verbal communication so often necessary in the doctor–patient relationship.

The Rodin museum in Paris, France, was also a great source of inspiration for me. The meaning of clasped hands in "the Cathedral" is universally understood, as is the angst in the hands of the "Burghers of Calais," and the tenderness in the embracing hands of "The Kiss." The diversity of human emotions expressed with and in our hands is legion. For physicians, the symbolism of "healing hands" is no cliché; indeed, a great deal more is implied in this term than needs explanation.

The disproportionate representation of the hands in the homunculus is perhaps the tip of the iceberg with respect to the relevance of the hands in human history. Romantically, I would like to agree with those anthropologists who suggest that the hand evolved before the brain. Certainly, the beauty, elegance, and finesse of the hand far exceed that of any other appendage of the human body. Is the hand slaved to the brain or vice versa? Despite advances in technology and science, as a surgeon in a highly technology-driven specialty, I continue to find myself at a loss to offer further technical interventions to some of my patients. For example, the young patient with the inoperable recurrent malignant glioma already treated with radiation and chemotherapy. In the treatment of such patients there comes a time when the scope of our intervention is reduced to holding their hands. Seemingly, when the latest tools of the digital age have nothing further to offer, the neurosurgeon is left with the ultimate test of manual dexterity: silent communication of compassion, empathy, reassurance, and prayer through the hands. For physicians, this kind of communication transcends all language barriers, and its essence is in their hands.

I have yet to meet a neurosurgeon who does not understand the aesthetic, physical, and metaphysical nuances of hands. Thus, unsurprisingly, the response to the hand photography project has been universally positive from neurosurgeons. Professor Gazi Yasargil was among the first surgeons of whom I took "practice shots" during his visit to London, Ontario, as Penfield Lecturer. These early photos of Yasargil's hands were in color, very rudimentary in style, and taken over tea at a sidewalk café on Richmond Road. Several months later, destiny placed me in Little Rock, Arkansas, in pursuit of fellowship training with Dr. Ossama Al-Mefty and Professor Gazi Yasargil.

During my time in Little Rock the combination of robust financial support from Dr. Al-Mefty and the arrival of numerous neurosurgeons for the Eighth Annual Meeting of the North American Skullbase Society, gave a strong boost to the project. Dr. Leonard Malis was the first neurosurgeon photographed in studio conditions. Once the early photographs were developed, the project gained momentum. The vast majority of the photos were taken at various national and international neurosurgery conferences, to which my highly capable assistants Johnpaul Jones and Jeffrey Bowen brought all the necessary equipment.

After I left Little Rock, all the financial commitments for the next few years of this project were completely my own responsibility. In fact, I rebuffed potential sponsors because they wanted to commercialize the project in a way that would detract from the aesthetics of the photographs. Despite the lack of initial corporate sponsorship, the early photographs received critical acclaim, with perhaps the most flattering compliment paid them when they were exhibited in juxtaposition with thirty of Auguste Rodin's hand sculptures at the Arkansas Arts Center.

From the earliest stages of this project, I have always been sensitive to the fact that the work could never be comprehensive, and that numerous neurosurgeons would be excluded due to practical limitations of time, money, and access. While inevitably incomplete and subjective, the final list of subjects in this book does strive to be diverse. Among the neurosurgeons included are the famous and the yet unknown, the senior and the young, male and female, those in academic and those in private practice, the local and the international. To the numerous neurosurgeons whom I did not get to during this project, an apology is due. My interest in photography of neurosurgeons' hands will not end with this book, and I hope to continue this labor of love.

FOREWORD

Through centuries of recorded history, the human hand has enjoyed remarkable attention, perhaps only second to the face as a representation of the unique element of individuality held by each being as well as the collective that is termed "humanity." Without question, it represents a special organ of adaptation and expression that is uniquely human and is frequently employed to "connect" elements of mind and thought to our environment, conveying and implementing ideas, sentiment, emotion, and the spectrum of human passion from anger and love to appreciation and gratitude. It is used to control, ordain, exert commission, praise, bless, harm, and heal.

Within the Bible's New Testament, numerous references are made to the "laying on hands" both by Christ and his apostles to affect healing (Luke 4:40, Acts 28:8), and ordaining to principle (Timothy 5:22, 2 Timothy 5:22) and purpose. Through such references in the arts and literature, and through legend and reality, the human hand has acquired mythical status. It has come to be an important symbol in each sector of life's specializations, but particularly in certain fields such as that of the fine artist, the musician, the athlete, and especially the surgeon, as it would appear to be the surgeon's principle tool for conveying the potential gift of life and good health.

The craft of neurological surgery represents one of civilization's most elevated and unique professions, and arguably one of its highest attainments to this point in time. Those who practice this skill, science, and art appreciate that it is the surgeon's mind and character that are the primary implements in facing neurological disease. However, there is a certain intangible quality to the facts of mind and character. It is the surgeon's hands that represent the physical embodiment of mind and the tool for implementation of concept and character. Each is physically unique and presents a concrete presence of ephemeral qualities, mystical and perhaps real, that are the essence of the historical human condition and our own genetic memories.

Given these facts, the artistic study of hands of individual surgeons presents a notable and singularly poignant portrayal of a uniquely important element of mankind—physical and transcendental. This study deserves contemplation and appreciation both from aesthetic and philosophical perspectives, with each individual bringing their life experience to the interface as in any intellectual communion. Upon consideration, the inherent drama and substance cannot be over-estimated!

Michael L. J. Apuzzo, M.D.
Los Angeles, CA

ix

ACKNOWLEDGEMENTS

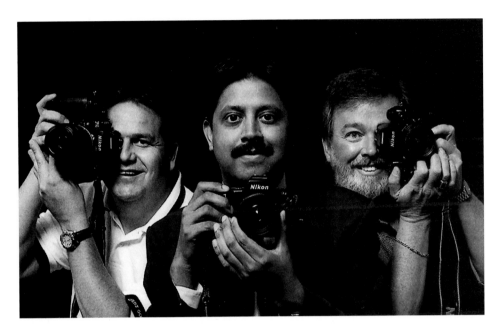

Jeffrey Bowen (left), Javed Siddiqi (center), Johnpaul Jones (right)

This project has been ongoing for several years, and my fascination with the hands of neurosurgeons is far from over. I thank the many neurosurgeons who allowed me to intrude into their personal space in attempts to capture brilliance, dedication, passion, and beauty. I want to thank my mentors, Dr. Gazi Yasargil, Dr. Ossama Al-Mefty, and the late Dr. Charles Drake, for instantly appreciating the philosophical and aesthetic merits of my work and for supporting it from the outset through to the current end product, this book. Dr. Mark Bernstein deserves recognition for selflessly promoting the photographs to my great benefit. Jeffrey Bowen and Johnpaul Jones started as my paid photography assistants and evolved quickly into soul mates on the same journey—I will not forget the warm glow of our effortless, wordless three-way communication in the shared pursuit of hidden nuances of shadows and light. Among the friends whose enthusiasm for this project continually energized it, but whose hands do not appear in this book, are: Linda D'Ascanio, Suan-Seh Foo, Larry Fortier, Catherine Hosage, Eugen and Elise Hug, Satish Keshav, Brooke Lawson, Moo-Hyung Lee, Tom and Madeline Lennon, and Simon Moore. I am grateful to my colleagues Dr. Chinyere Obasi and Dr. Timothy Wiebe, both of whom made many sacrifices to allow me the freedom to complete this project. My residents Josif Borovic, John Cantando, Dennis Miller, John Spitalieri, and Darryl Warner were also sources of inspiration for me. Many of the last minute items could not have been completed without the help of my secretary, Madeline Castorena, whose good judgement and sense of aesthetics have been important resources for me. Finally, I want to thank my publisher, Thieme, for seeing sufficient value in this work to venture into a first-ever publication of this type and for untiring efforts to see it to an end in a timely manner. I had wonderful help in this project and any errors in the final product are entirely mine.

DEDICATION

This book is dedicated to my father, Ishaque Siddiqi, who enjoyed many of the hand photographs prior to his recent death. It is also dedicated to my mother, Aysha, and my sisters, Shahina and Zarina, who see worth in all my efforts and who are my strongest pillars.

IN THEIR HANDS

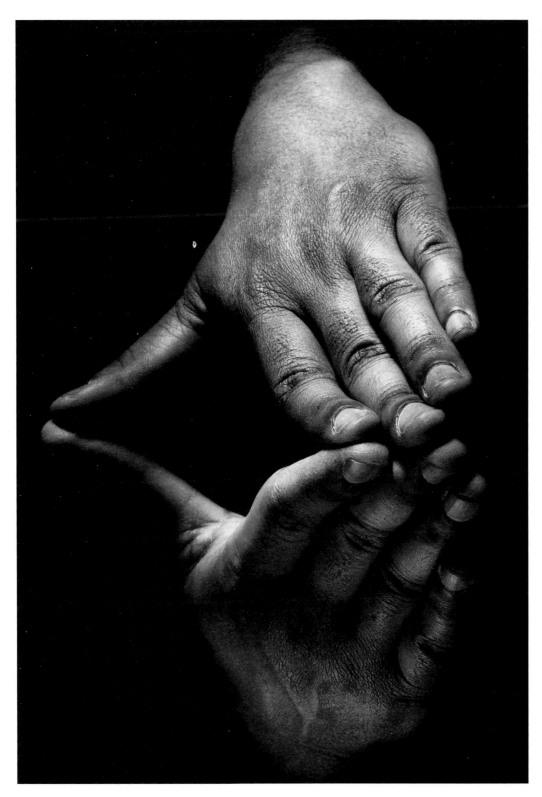

3

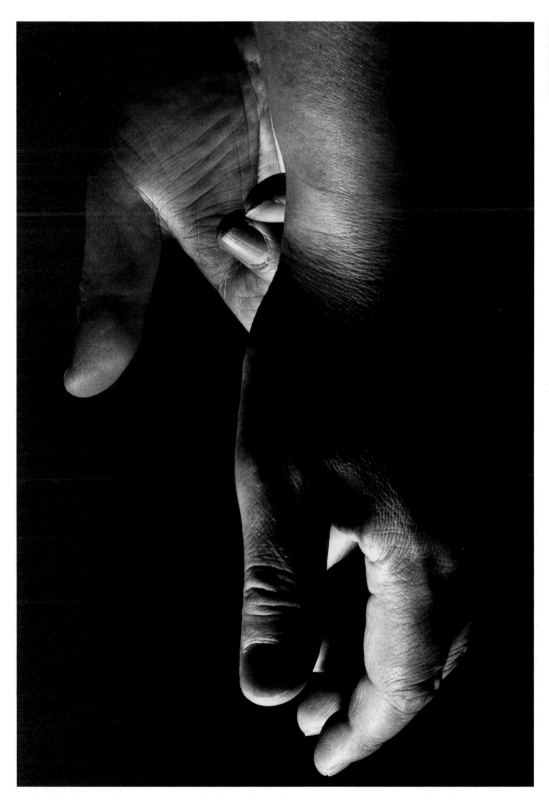

ABE, HIROSHI

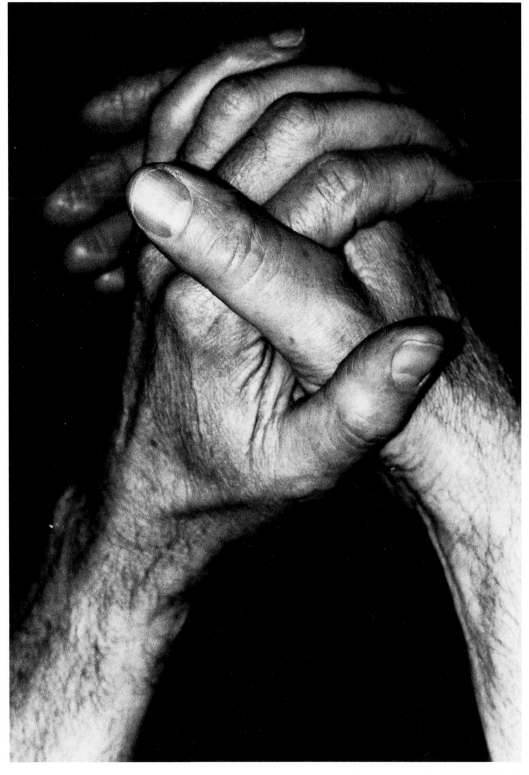

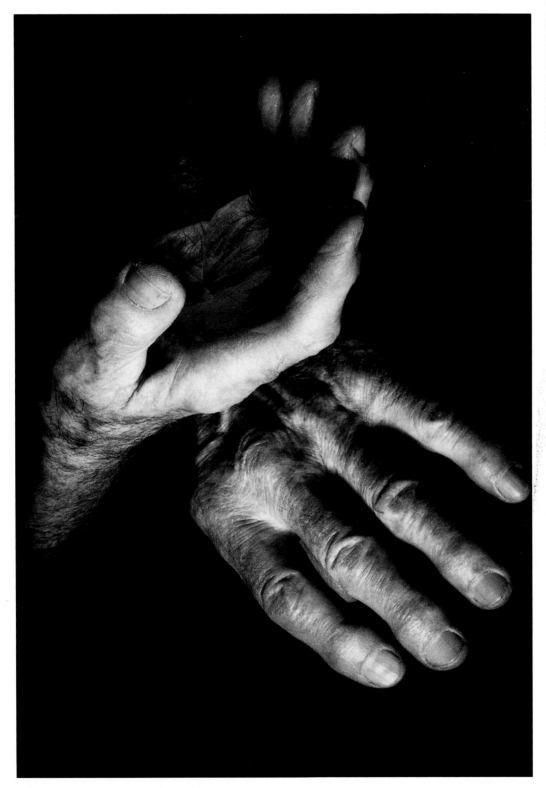

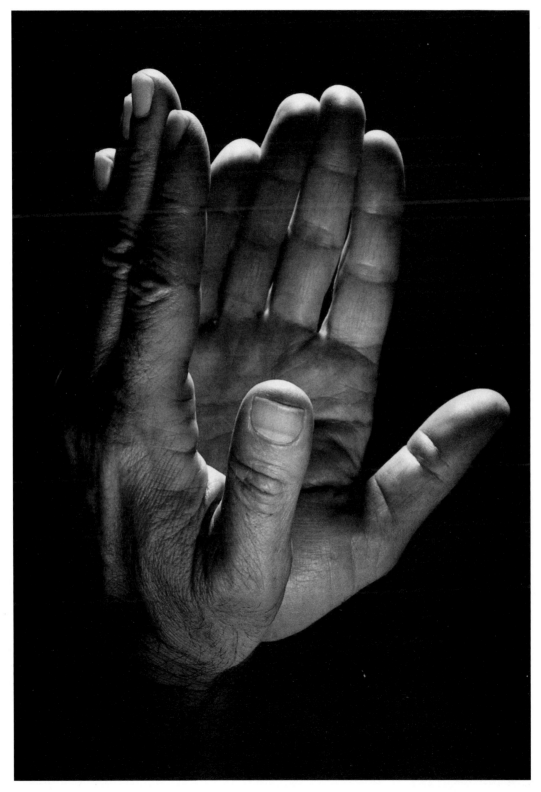

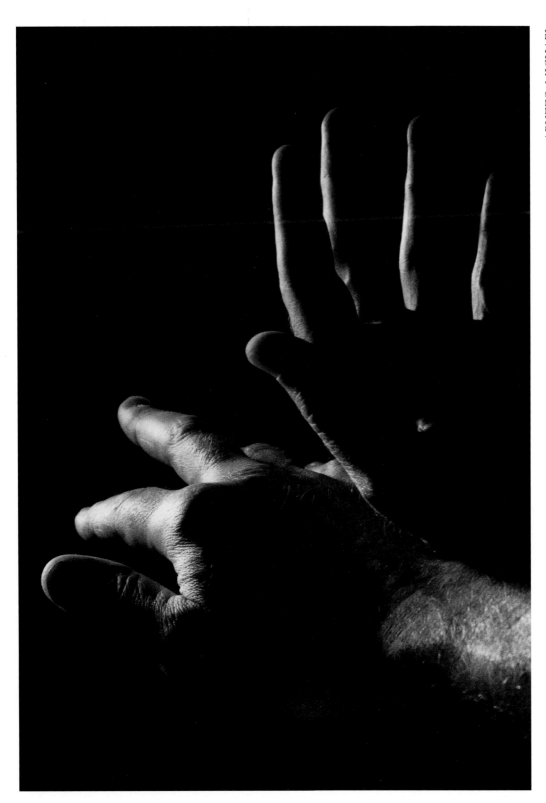

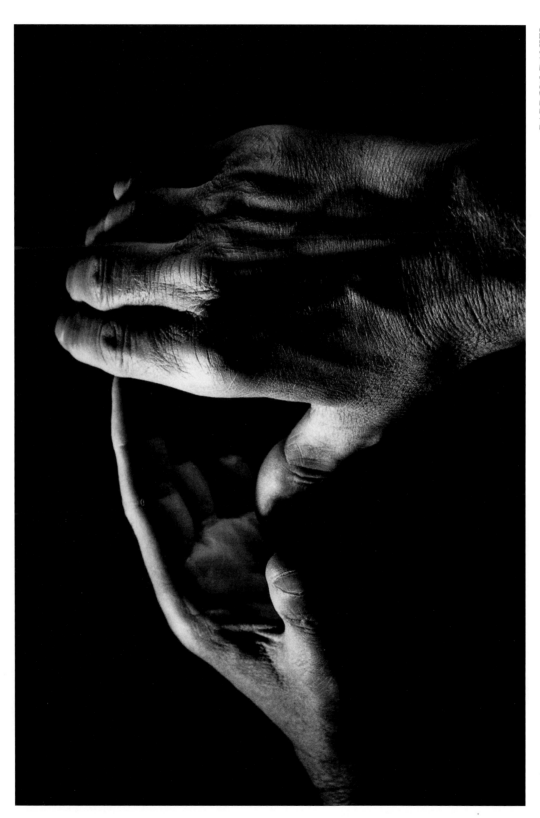

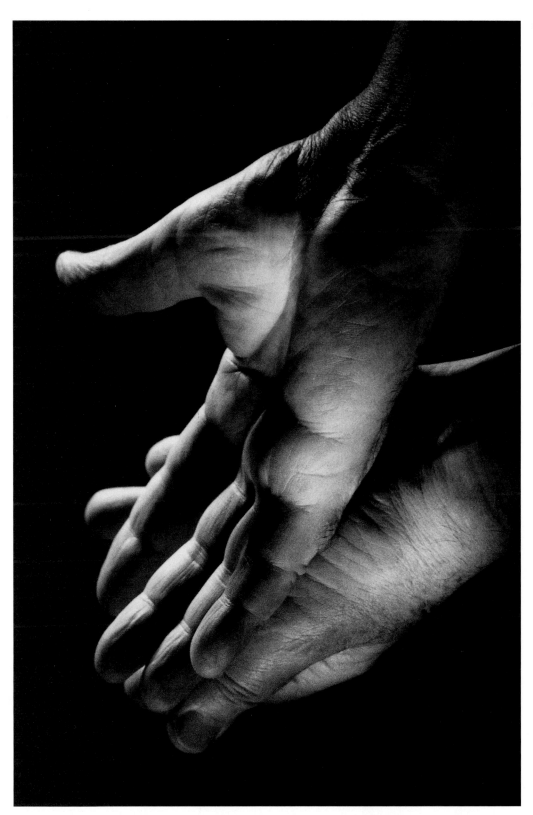

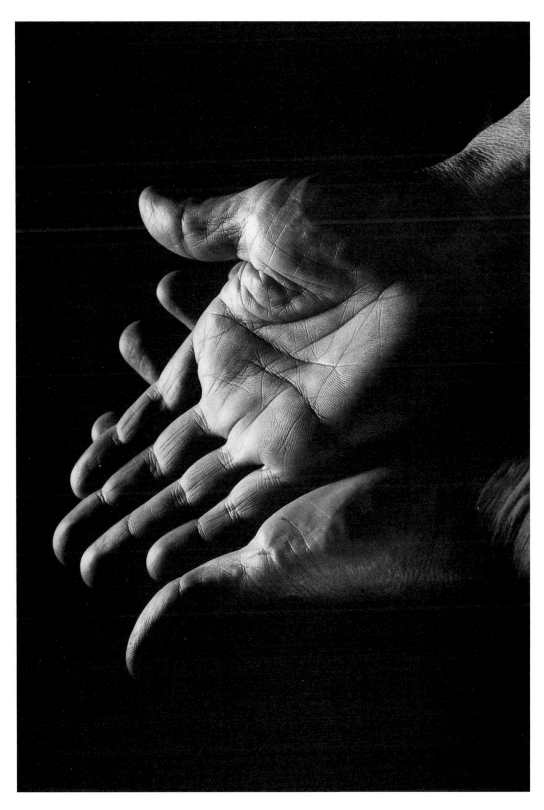

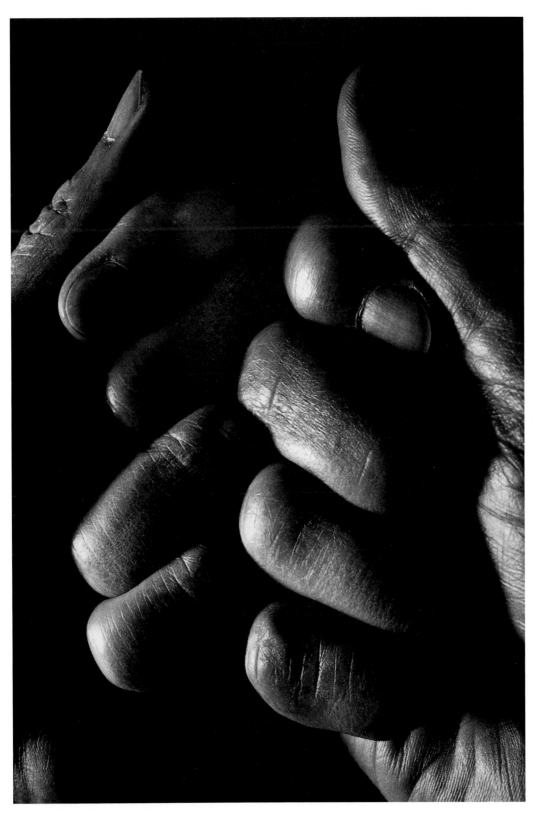

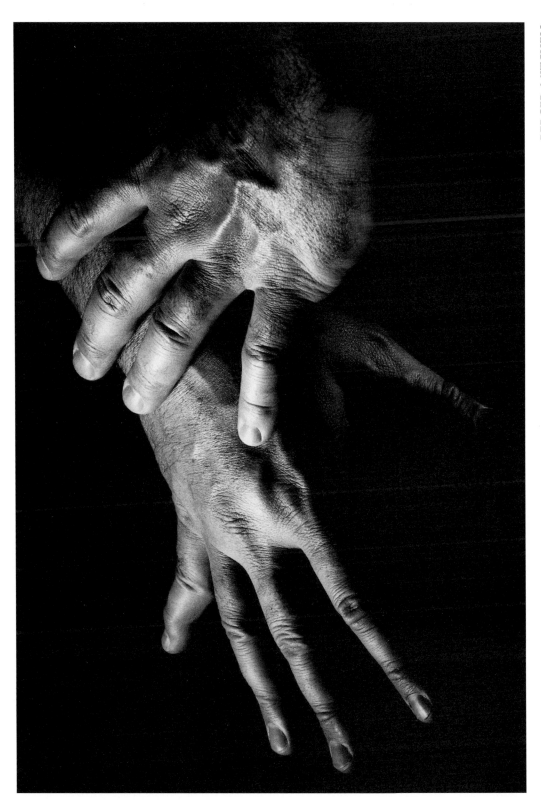

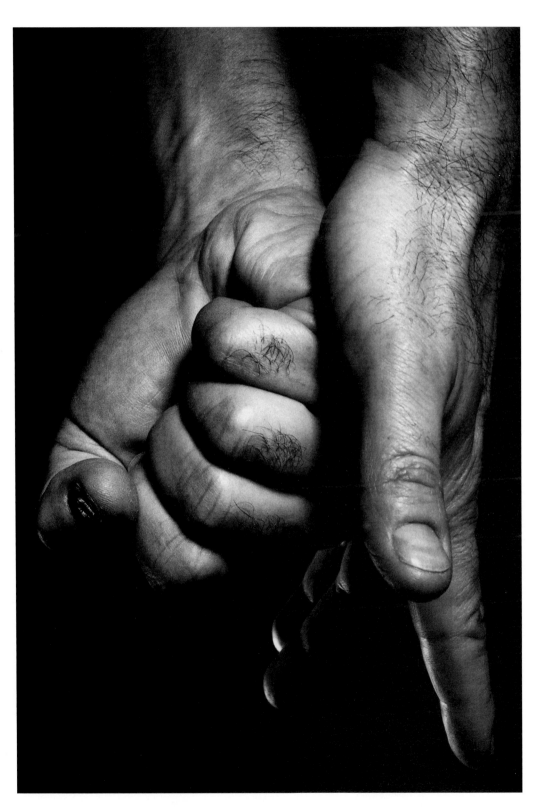

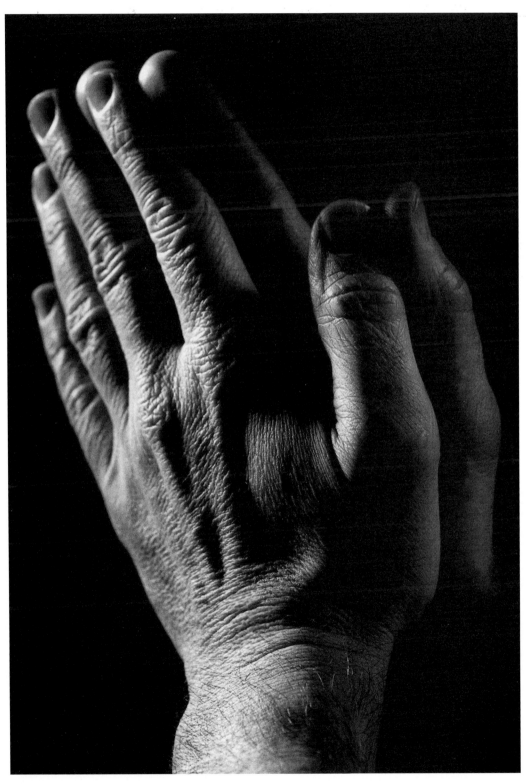

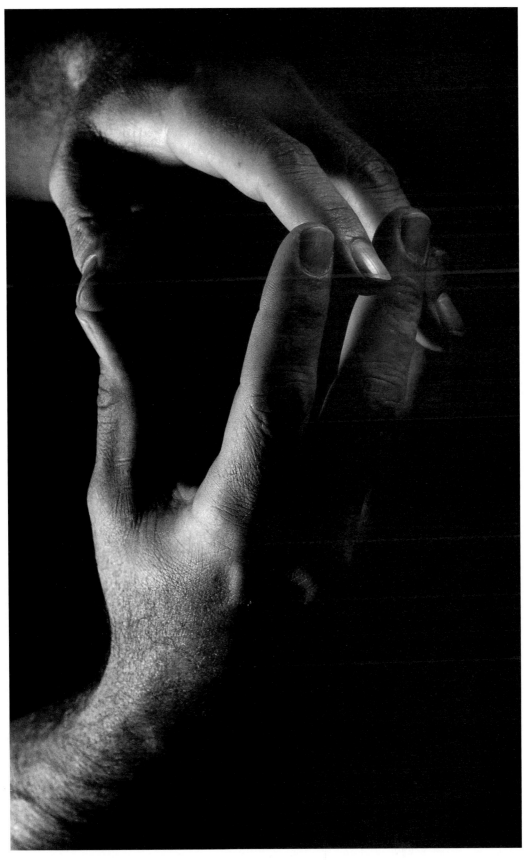

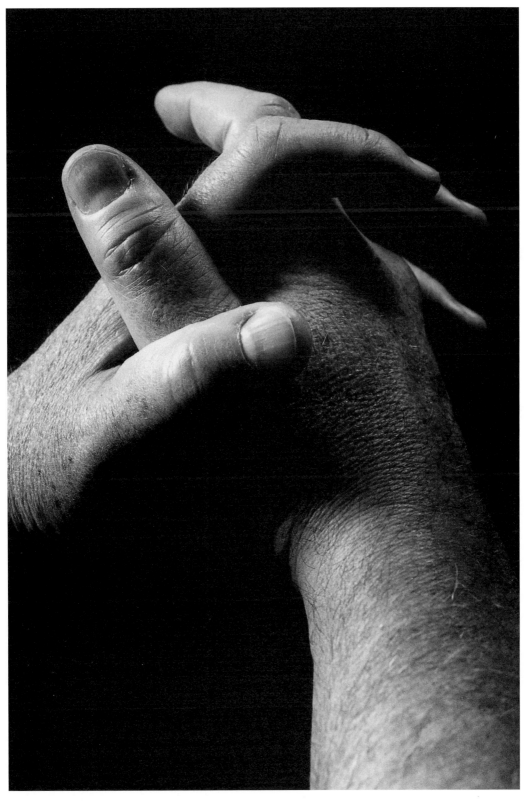

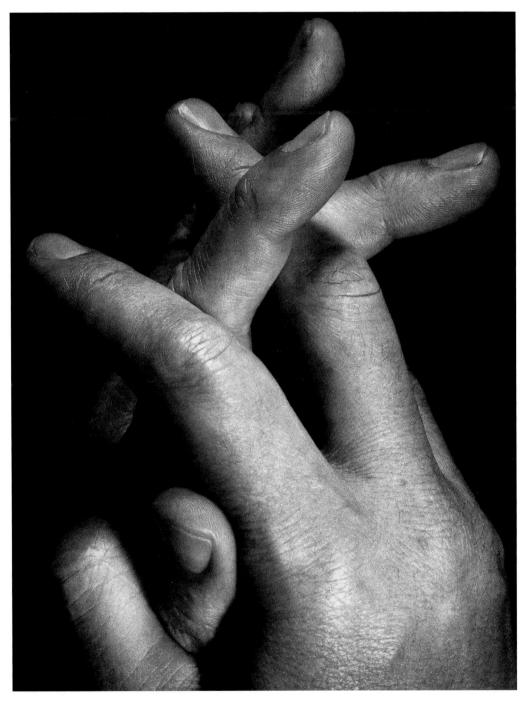

BUCHOLZ, RICHARD   *33*

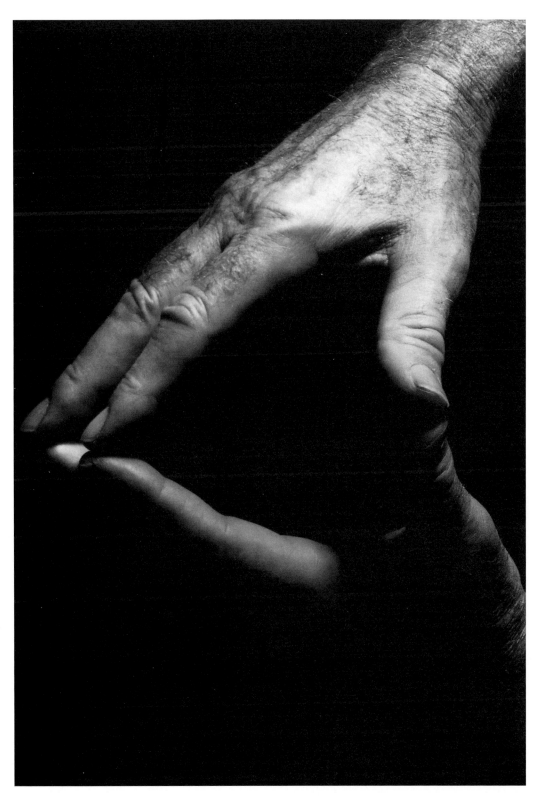

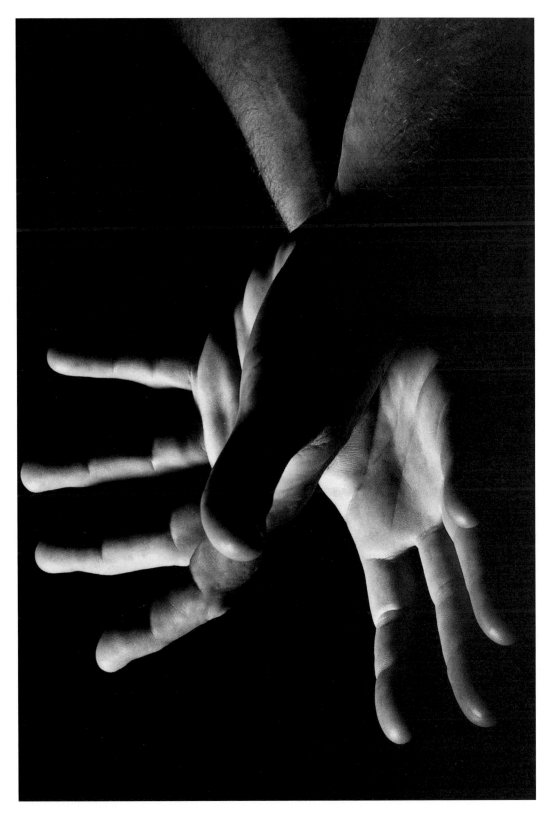

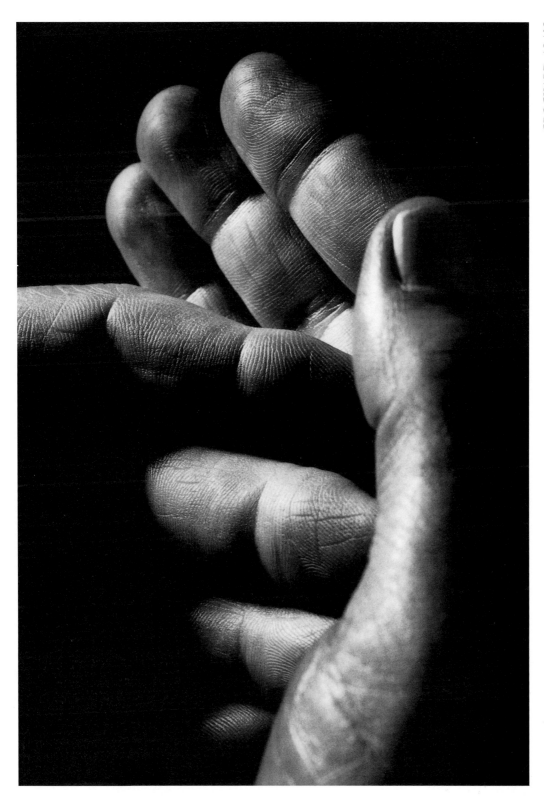

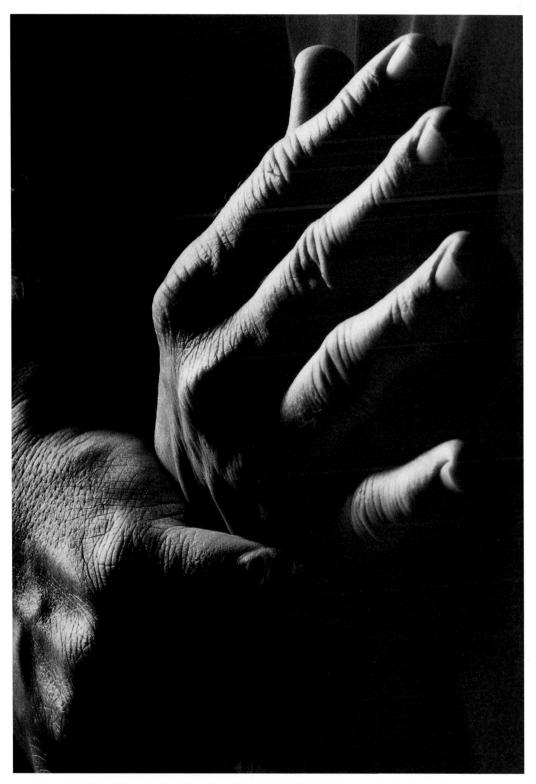

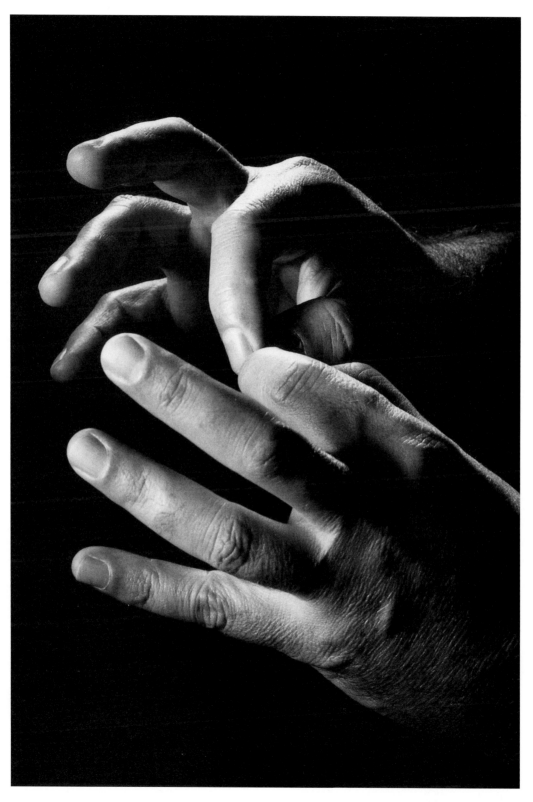

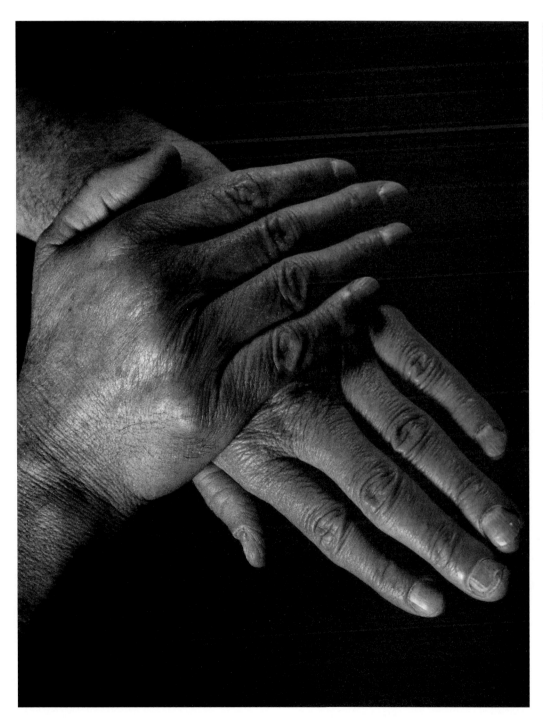

45

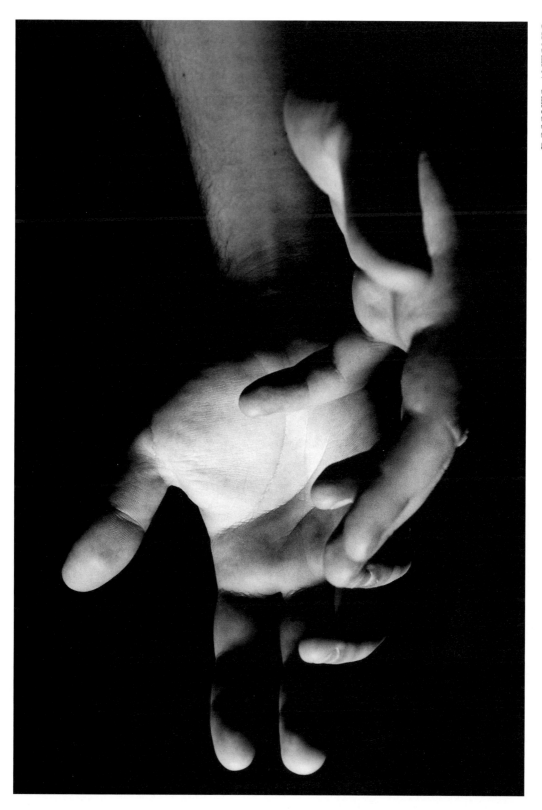

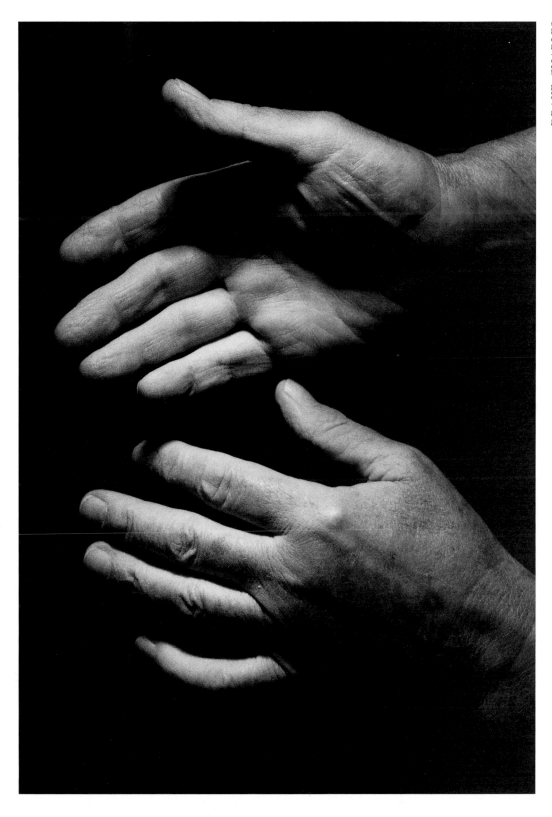

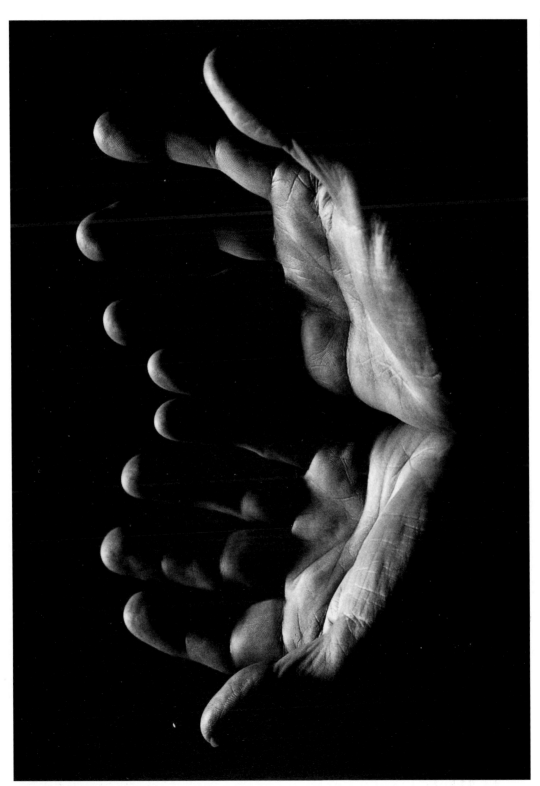

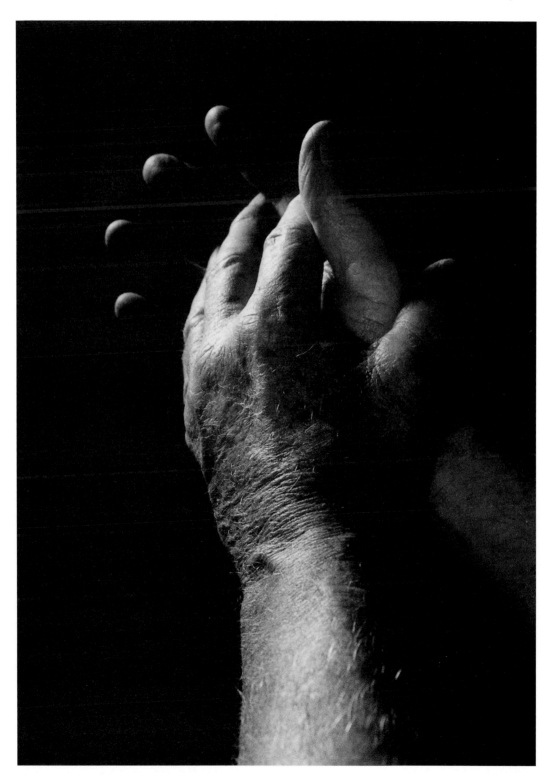

53

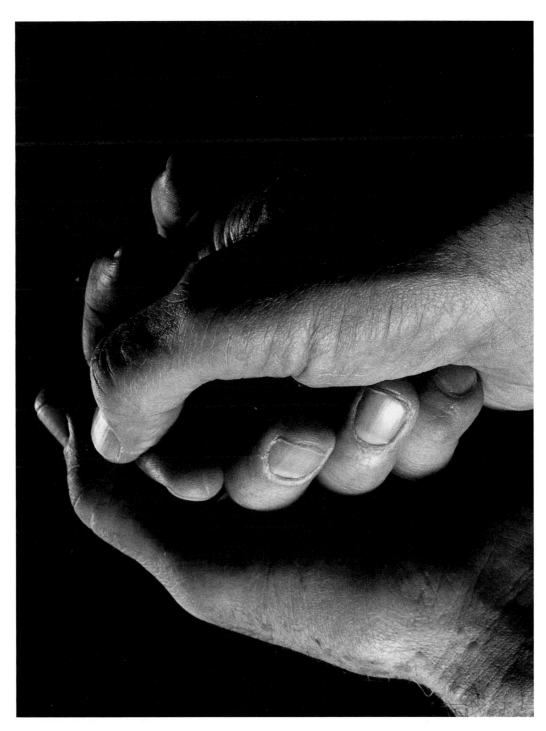

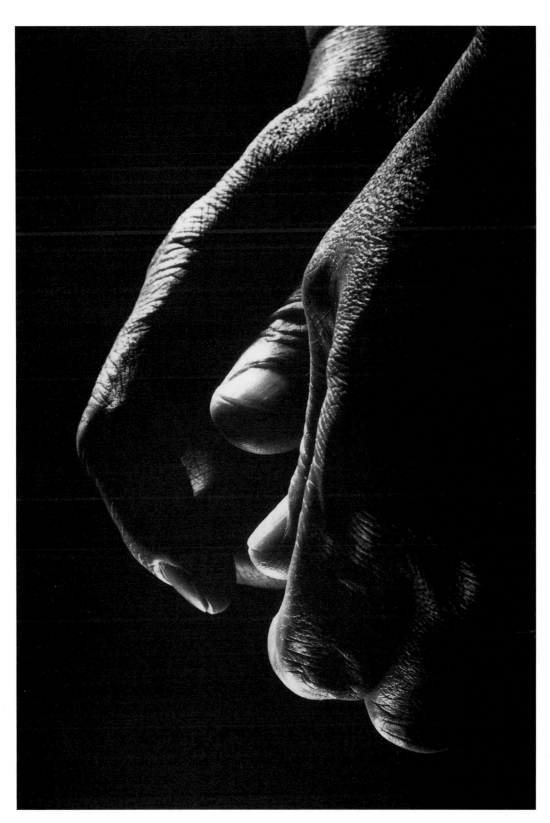

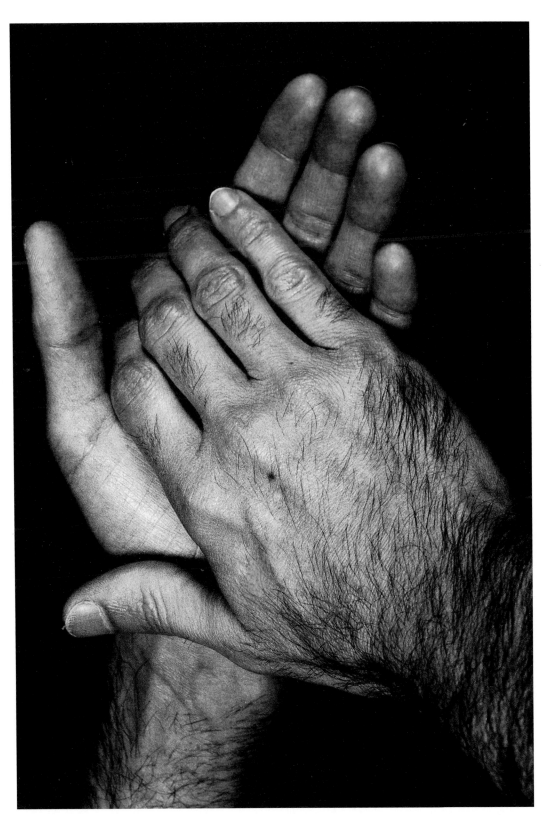

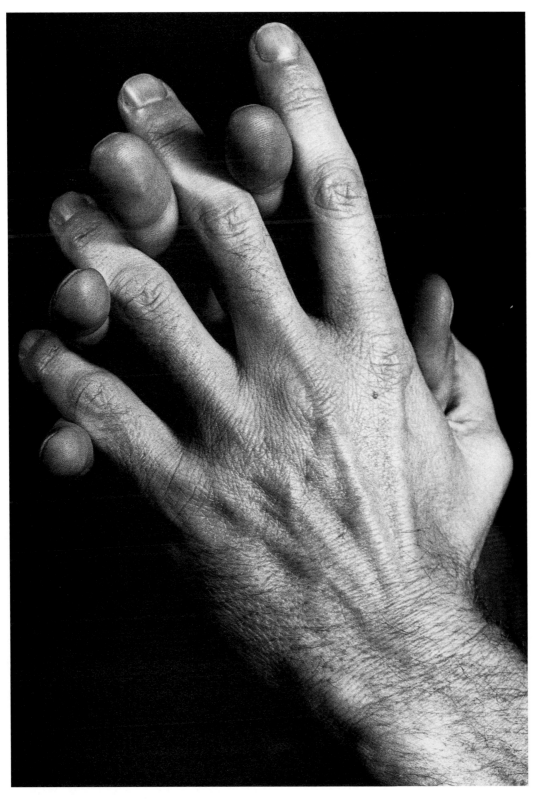

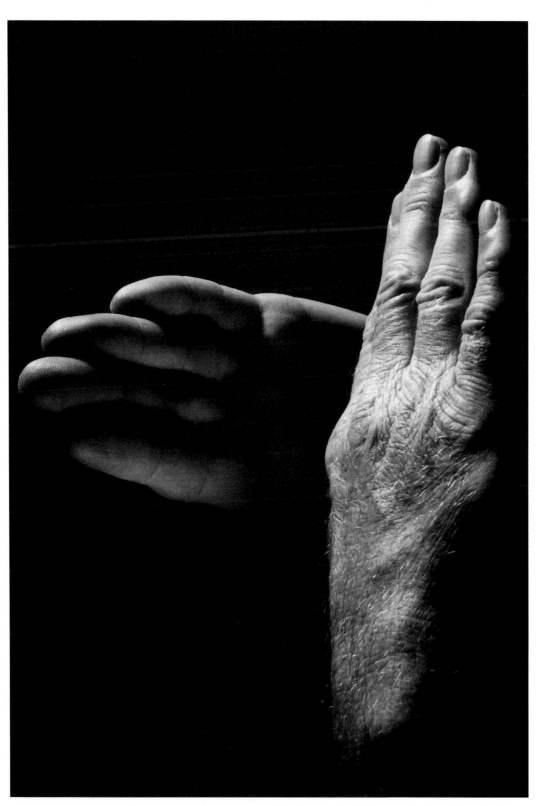

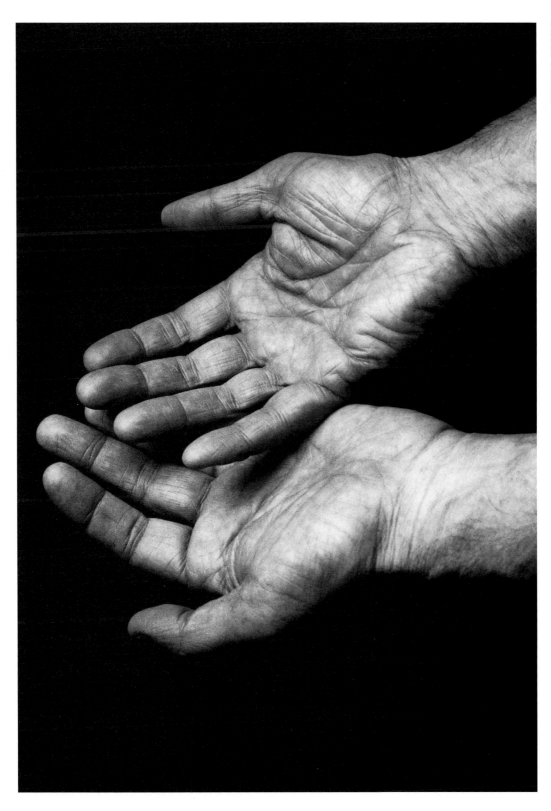

GIRVIN, JOHN

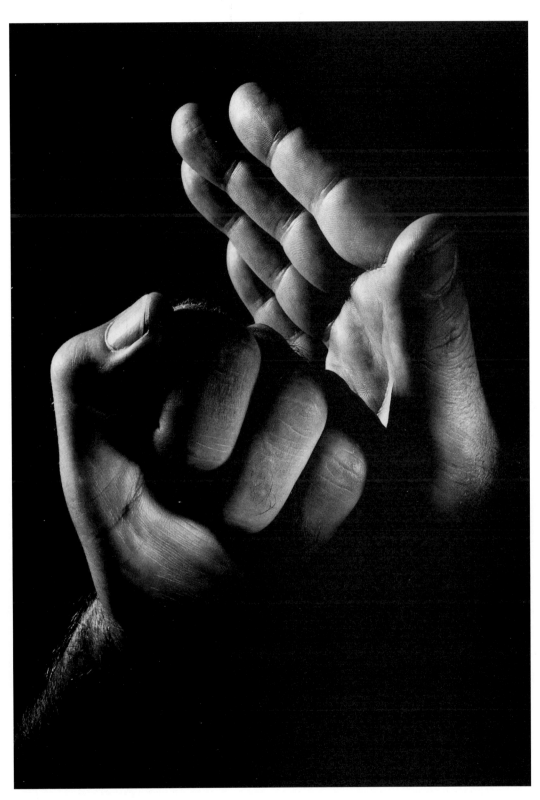

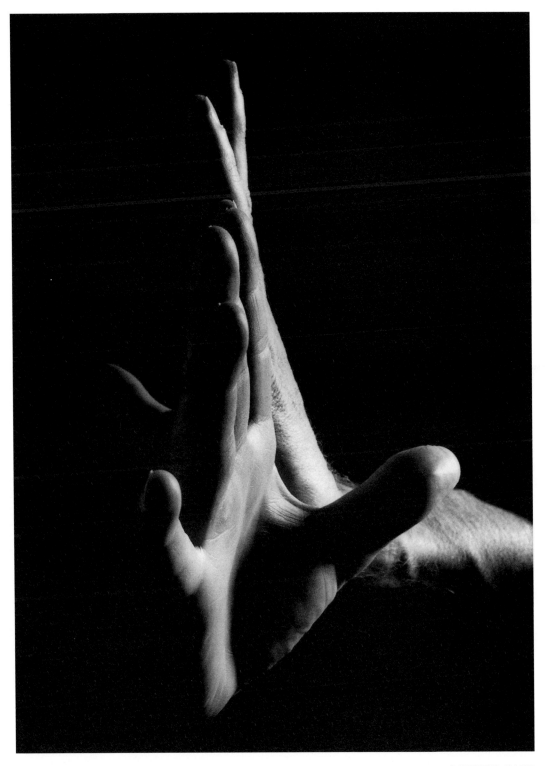

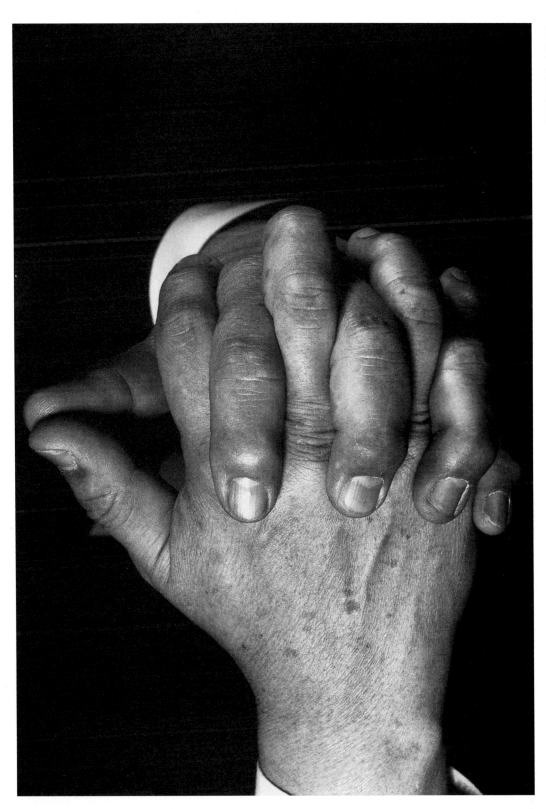

71

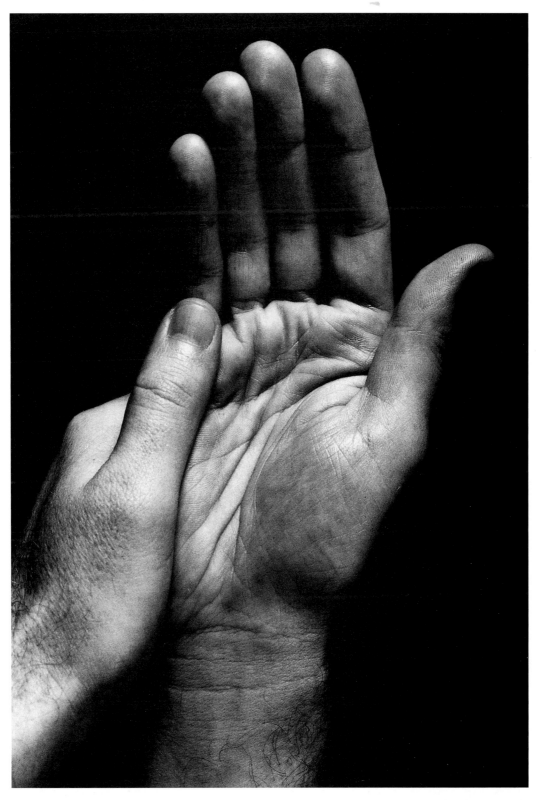

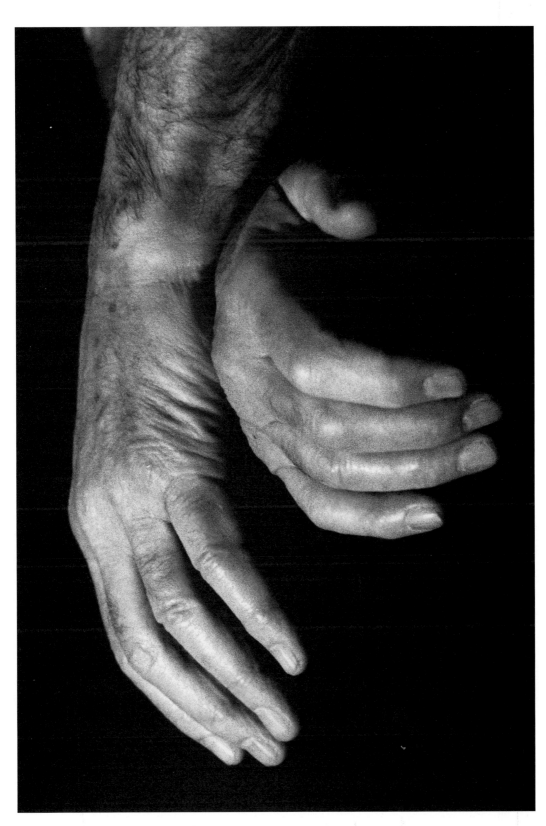

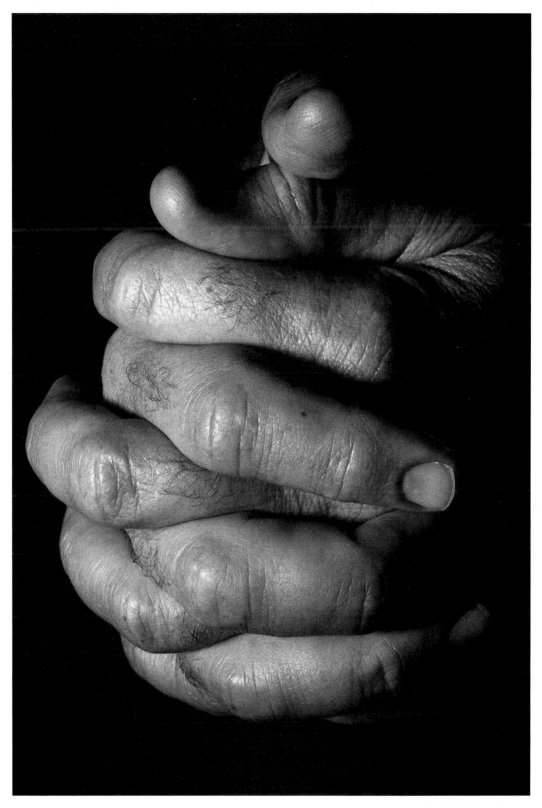

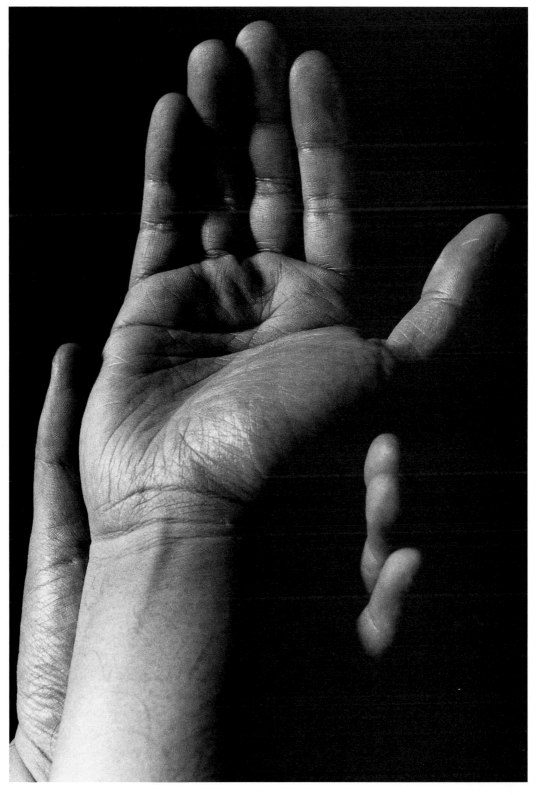

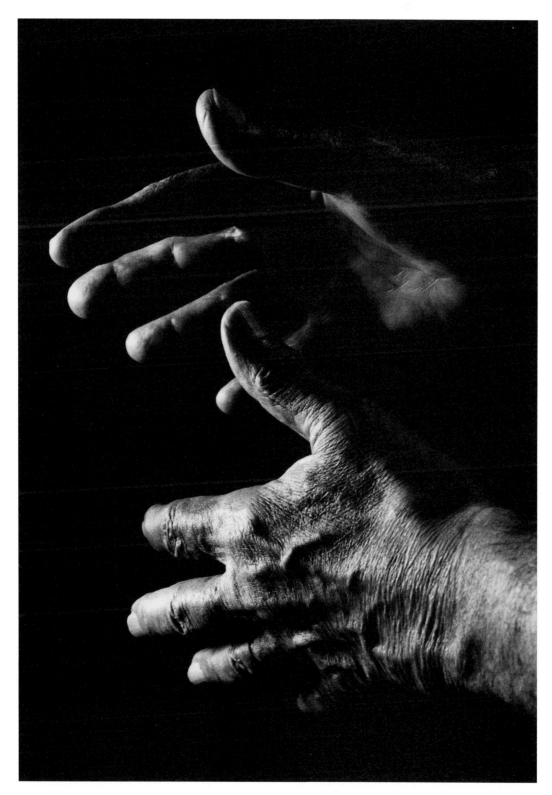

81

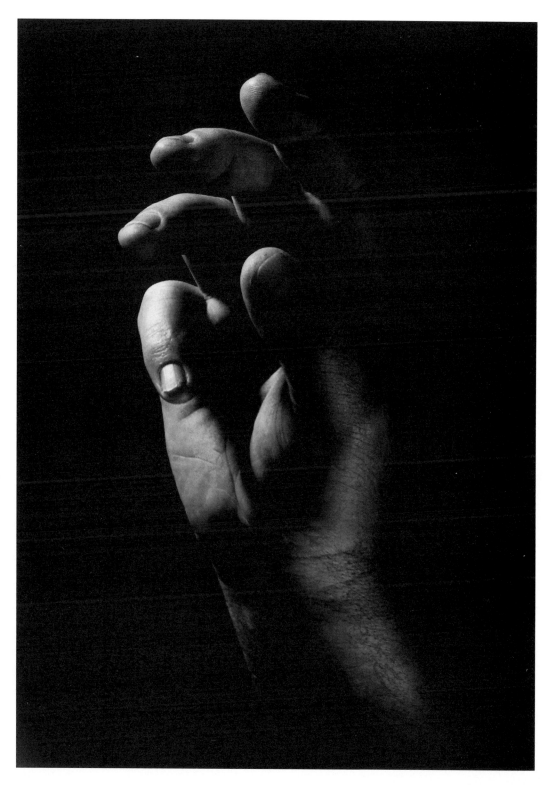

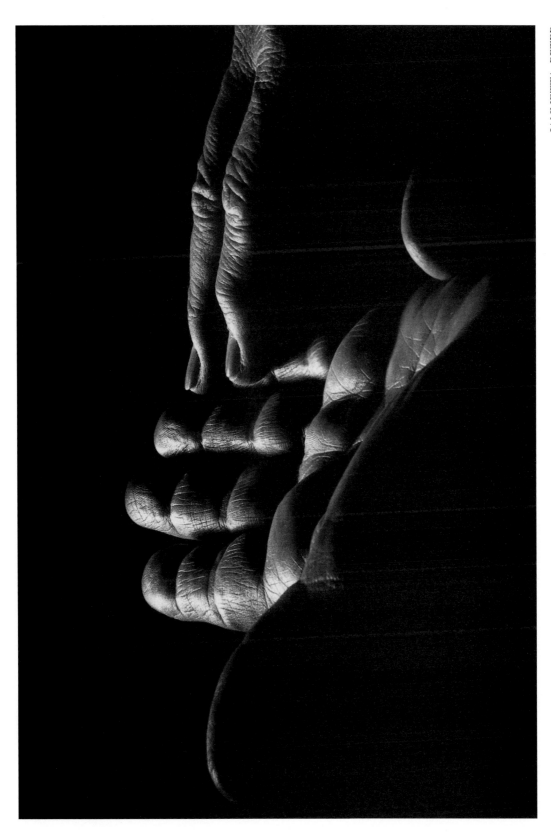

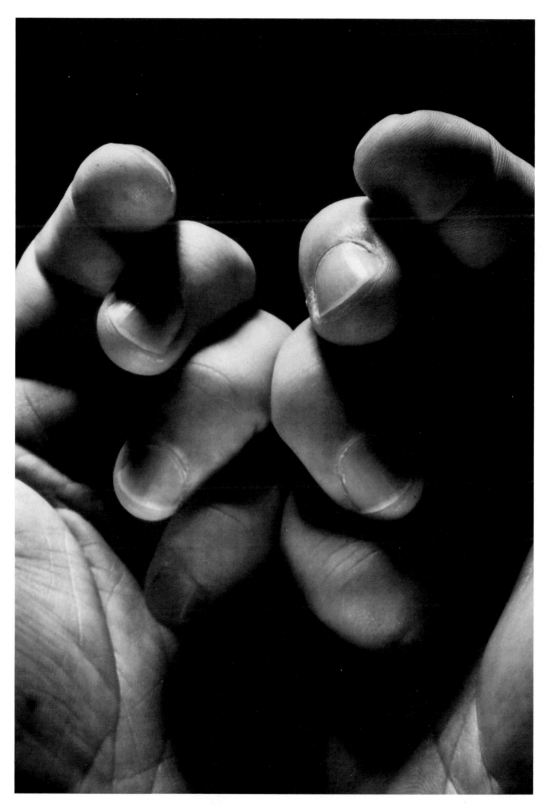

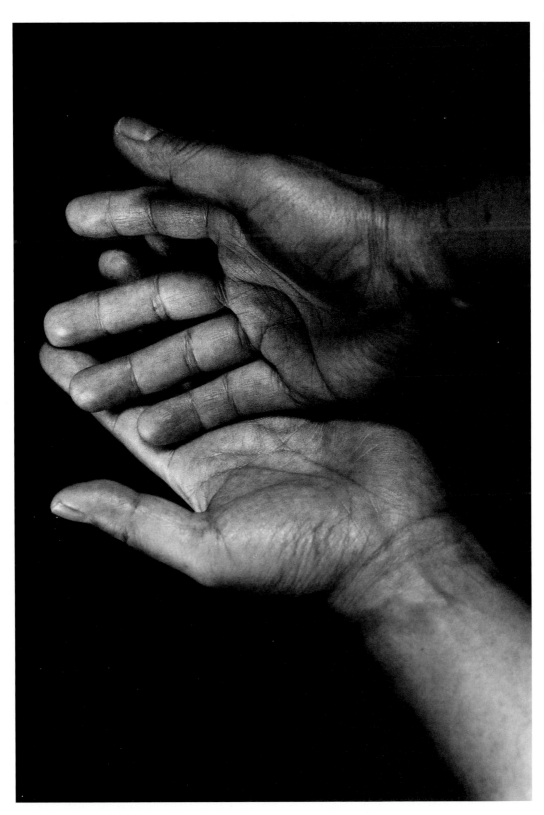

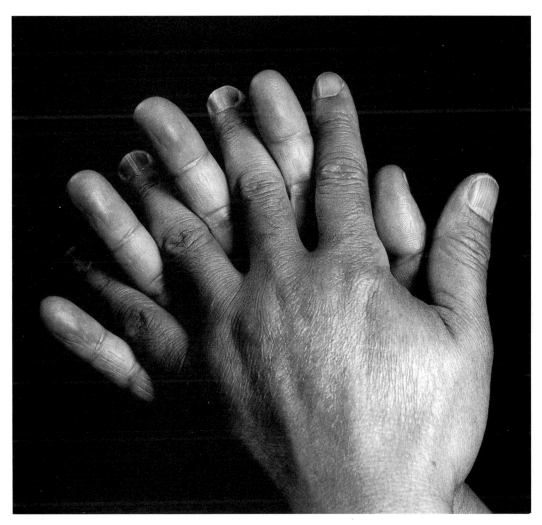

KAWASE, TAKESHI

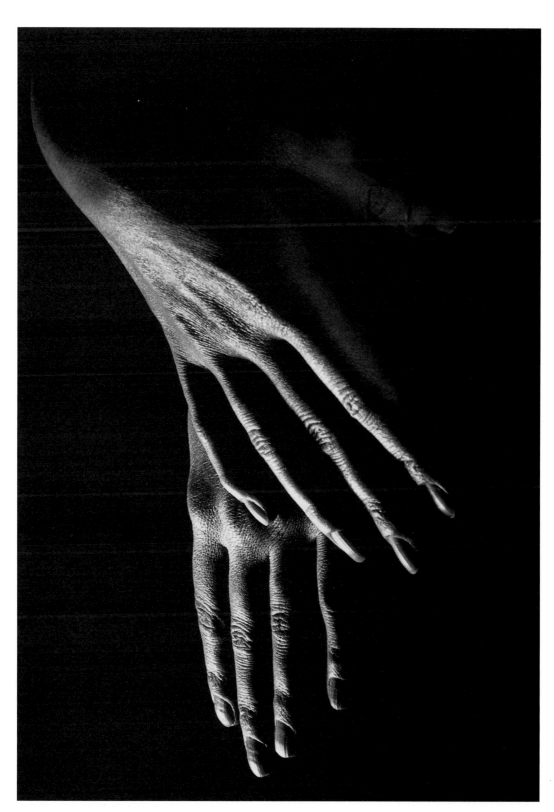

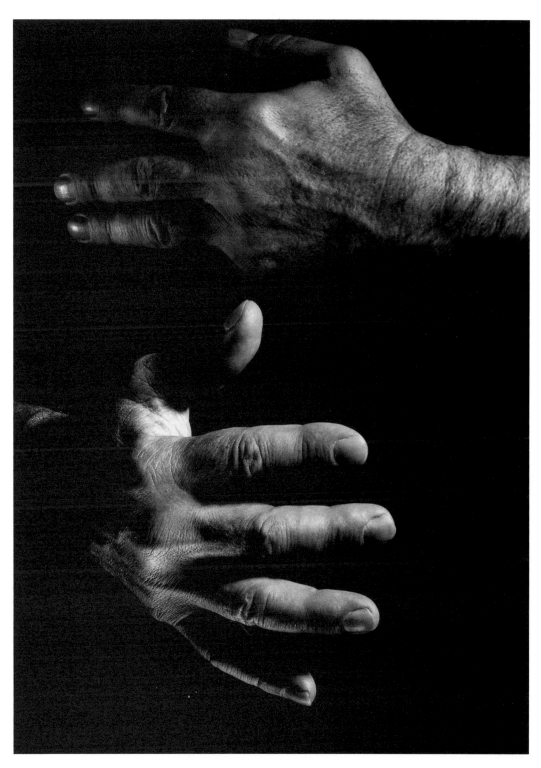

95

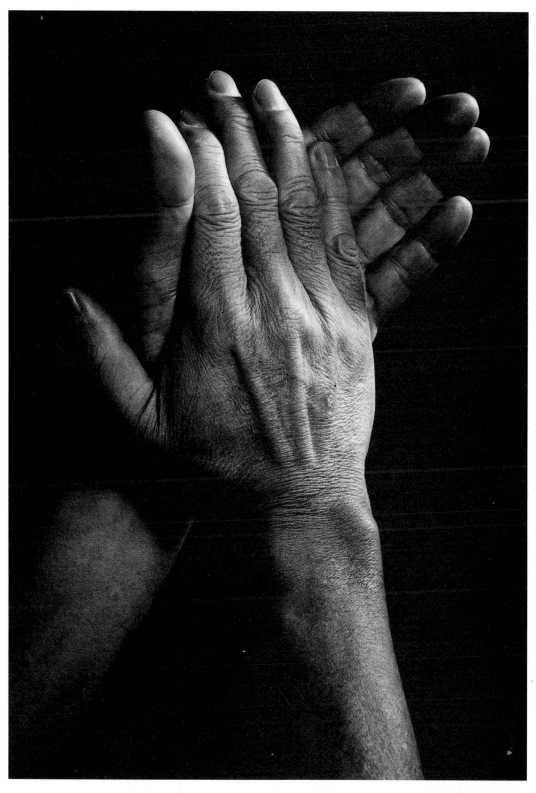

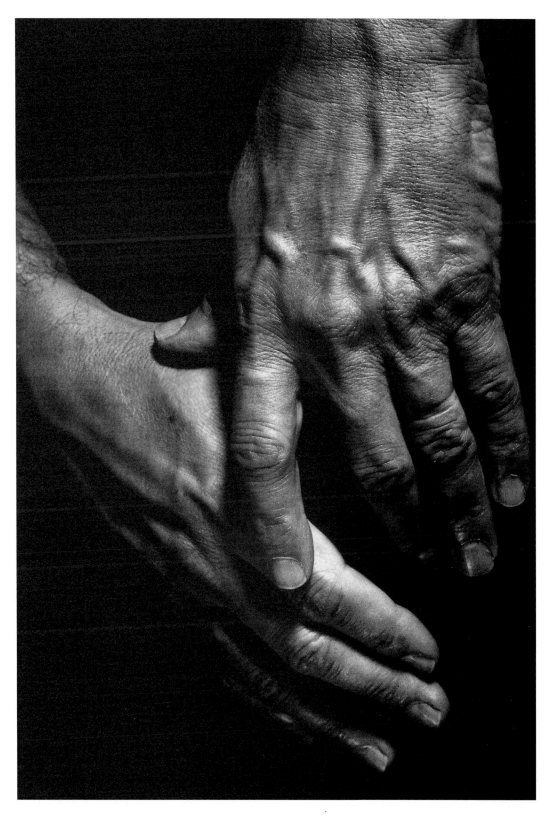

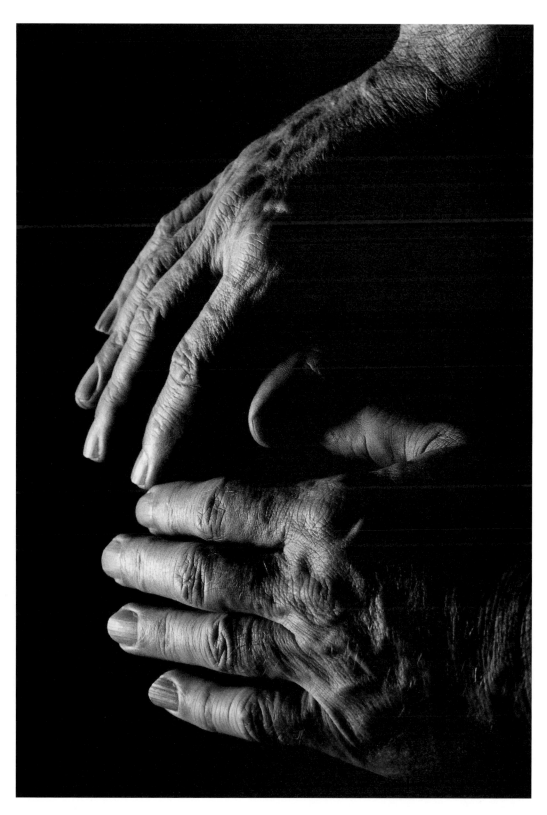

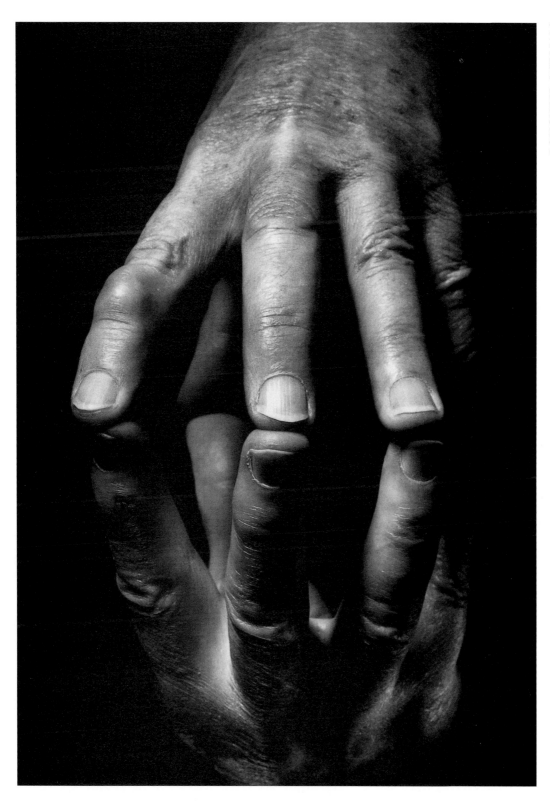

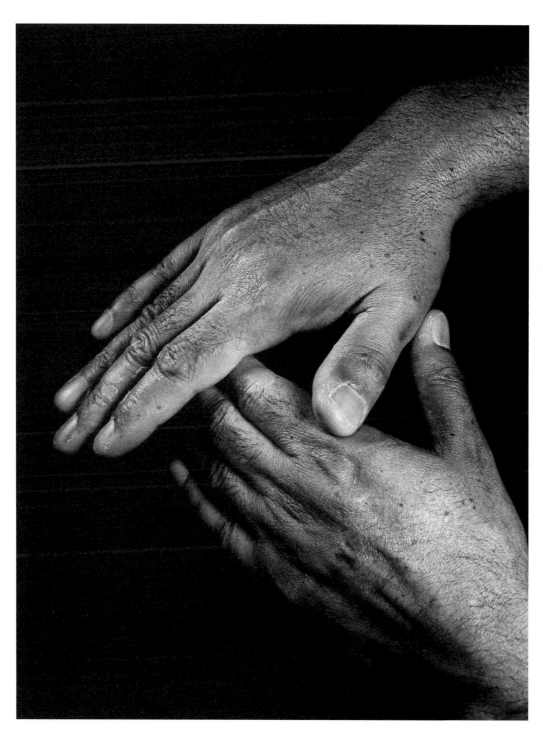

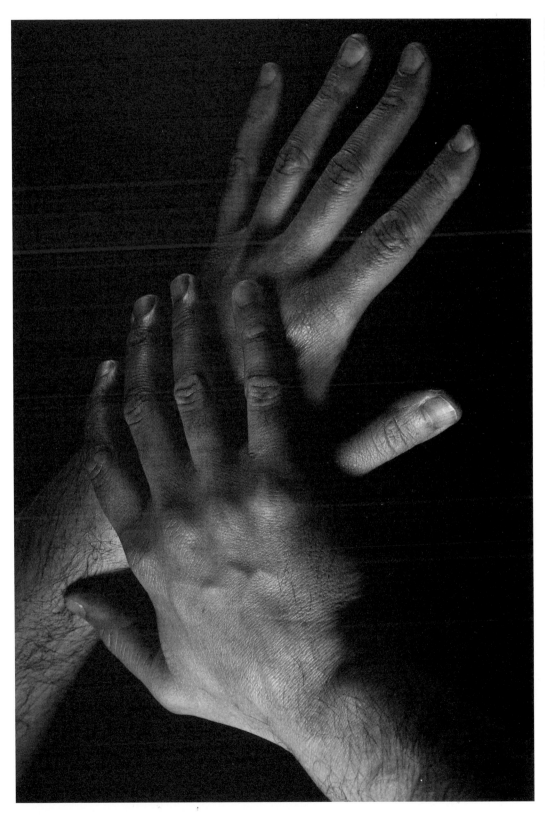

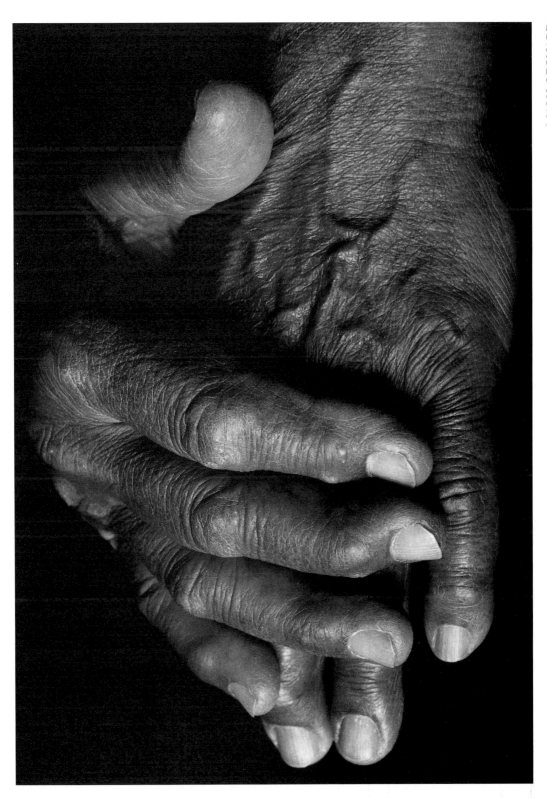

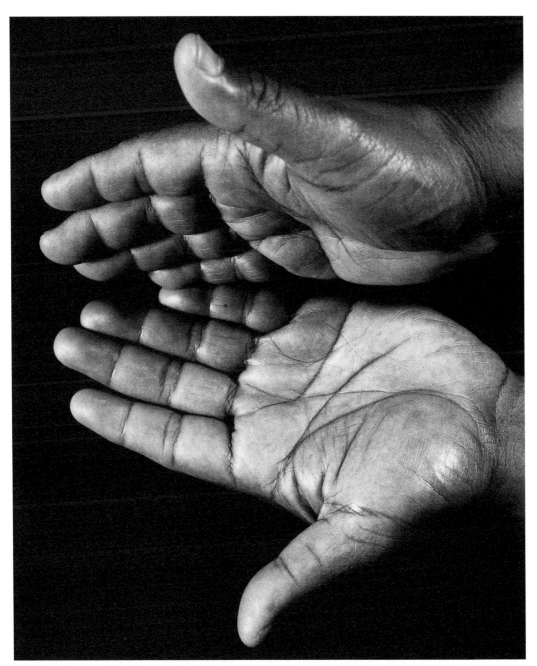

111

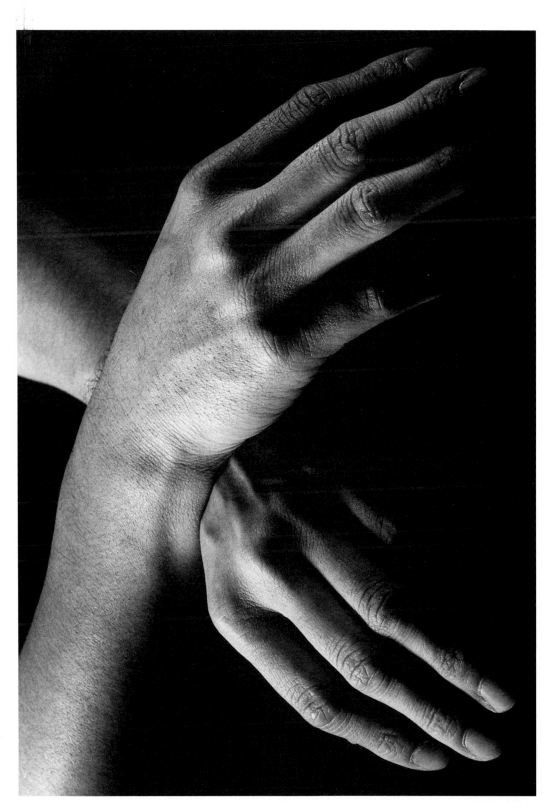

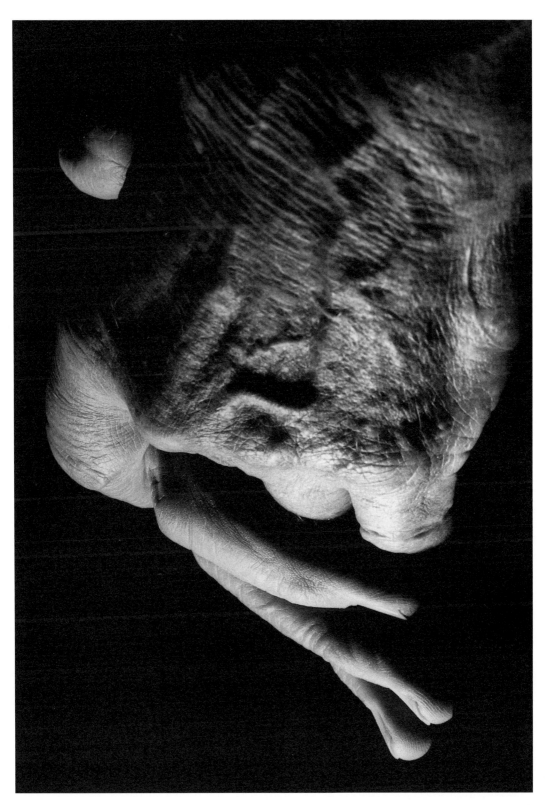

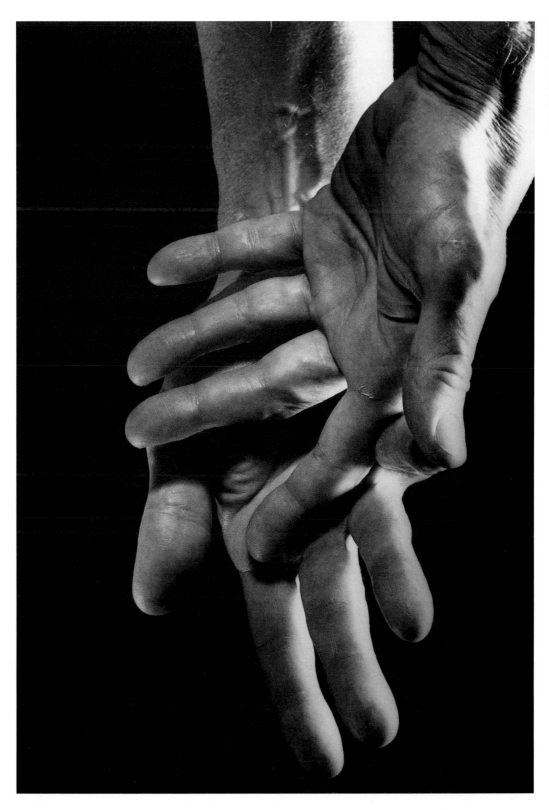

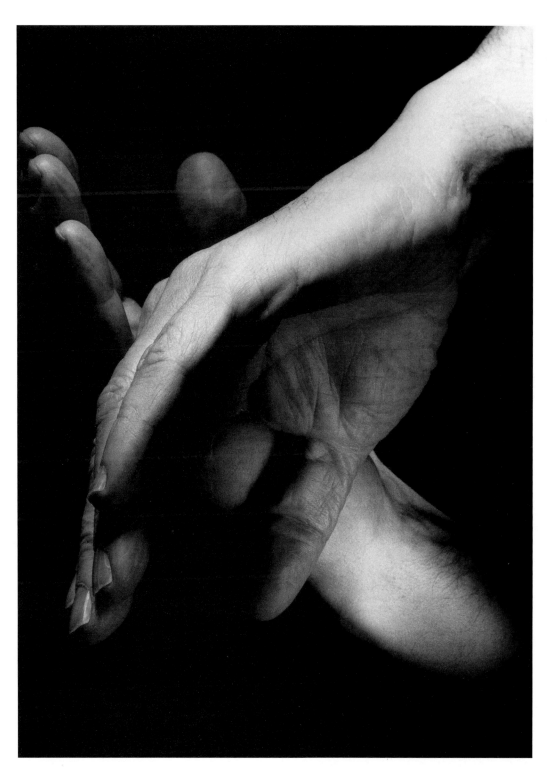

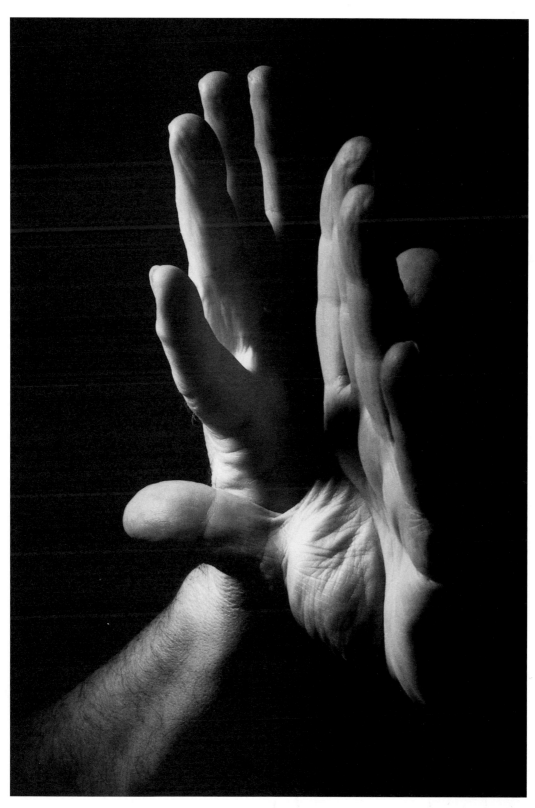

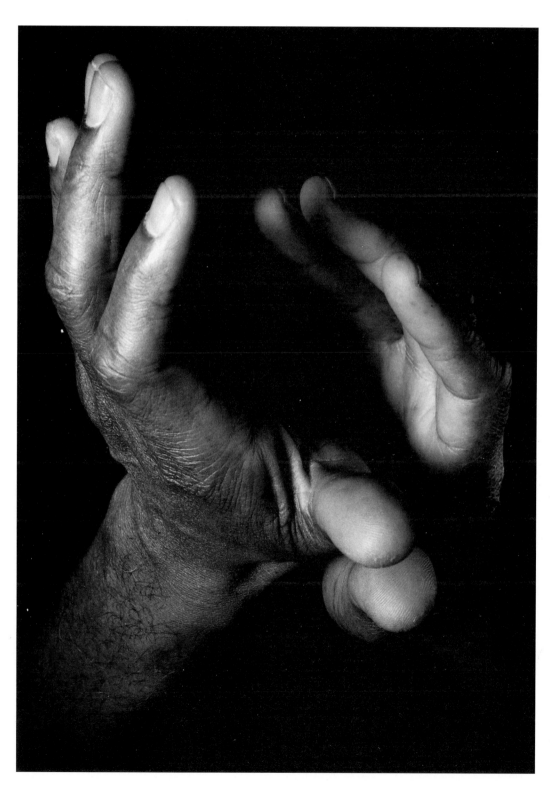

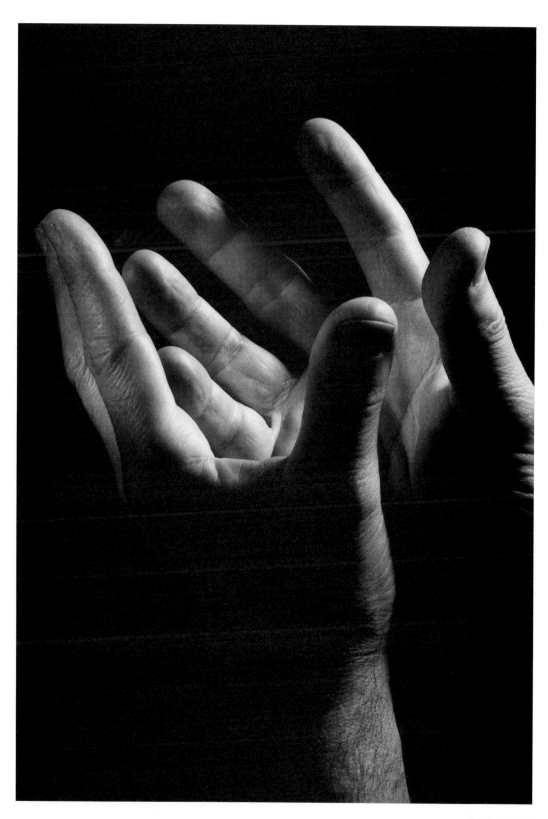

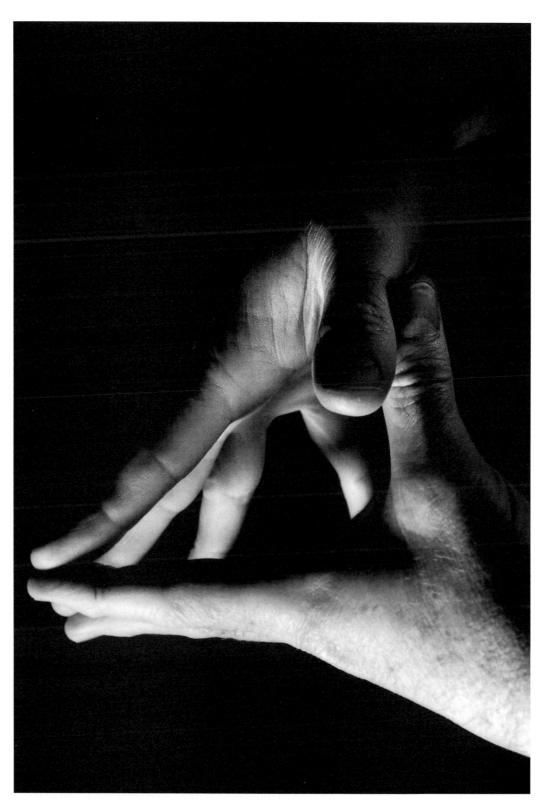

127

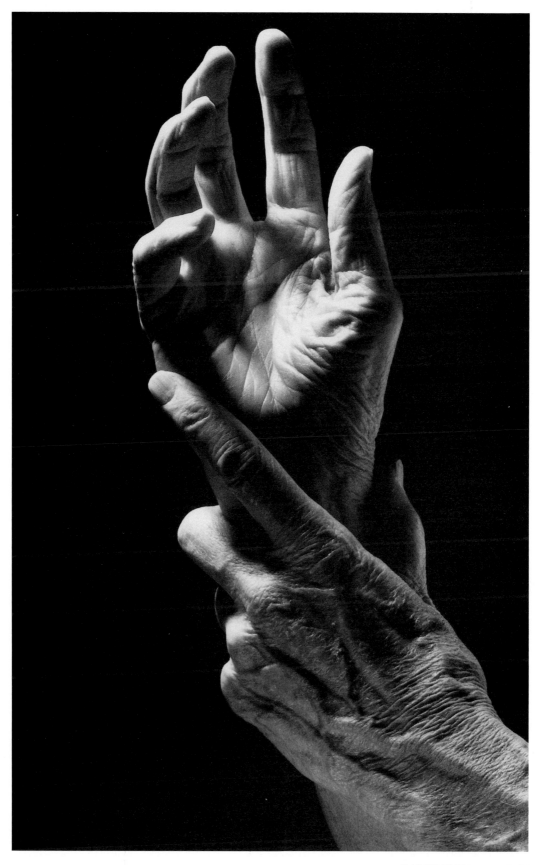

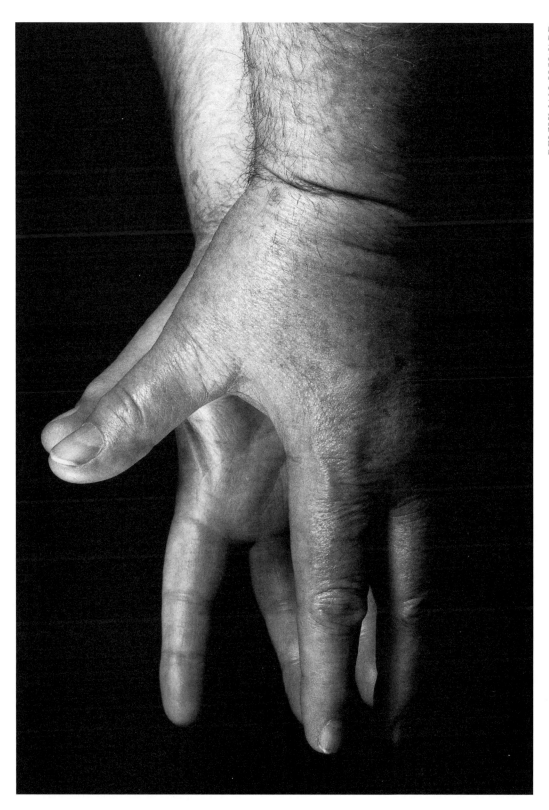

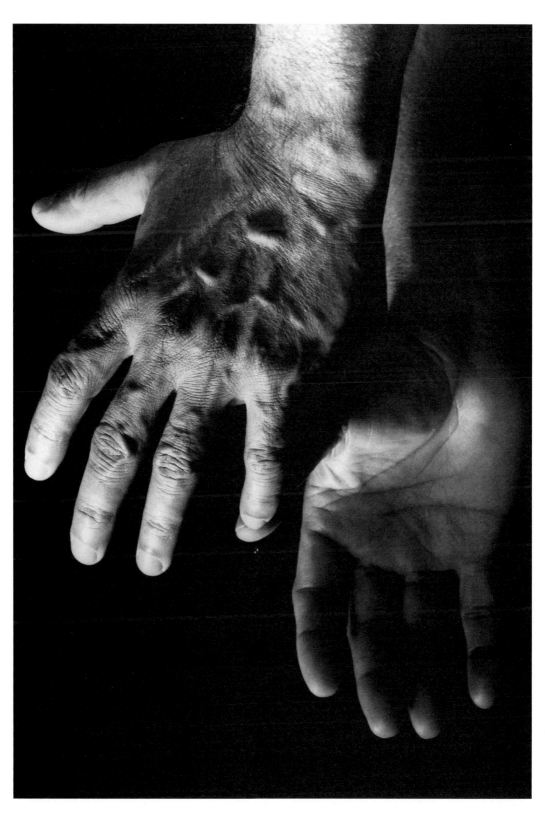

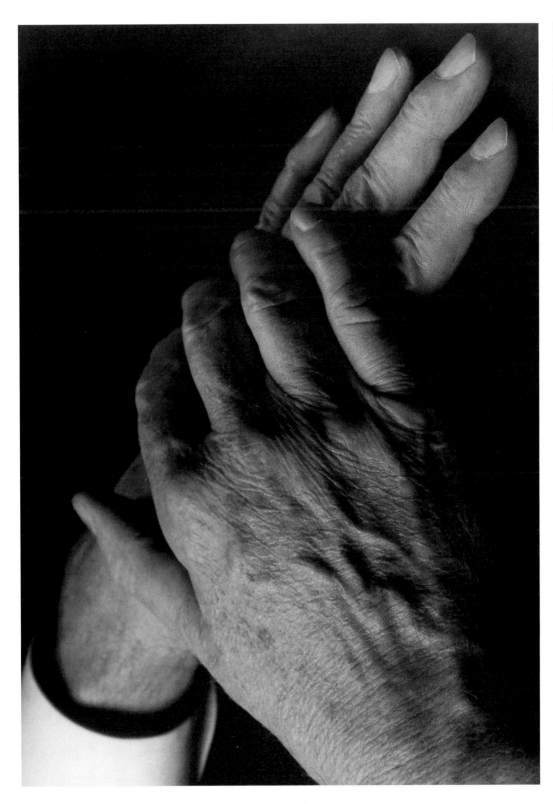

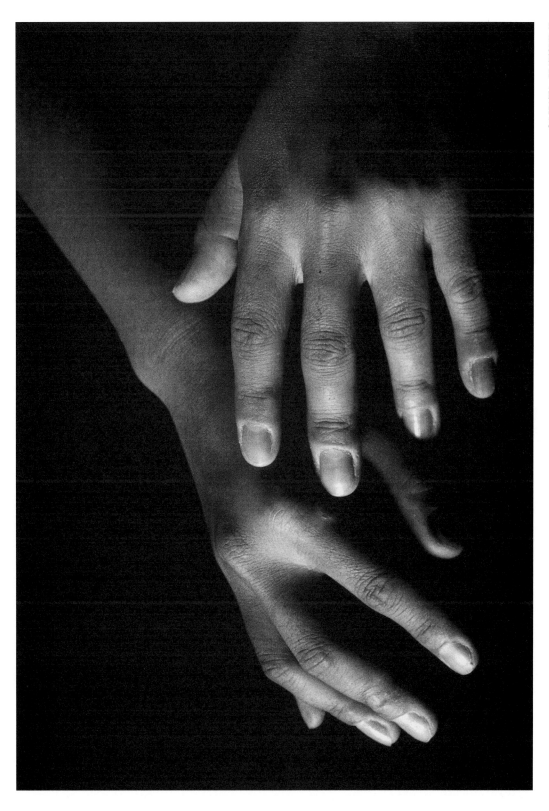

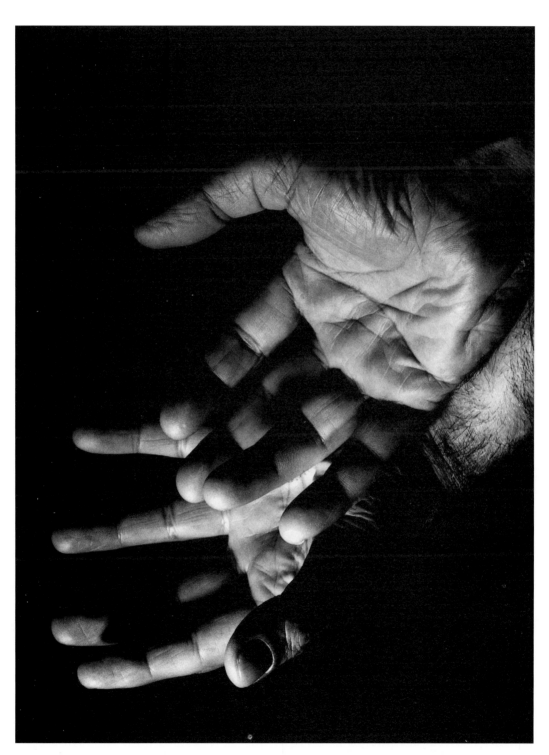

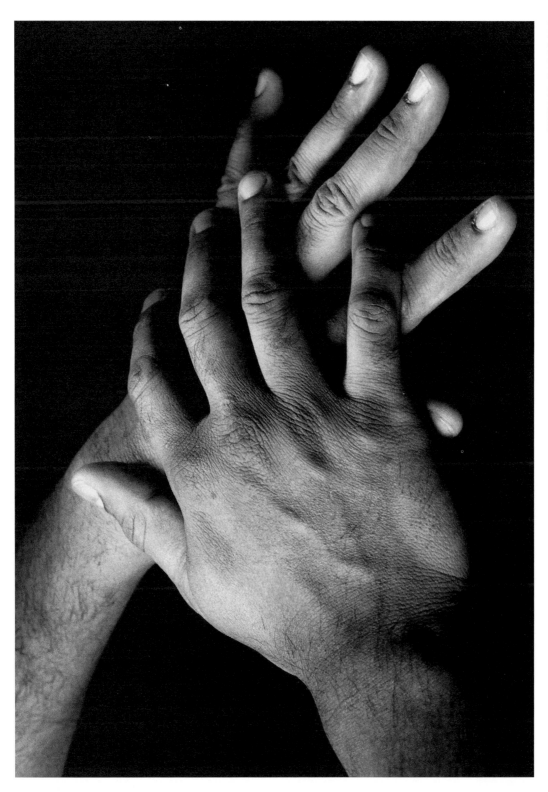

141

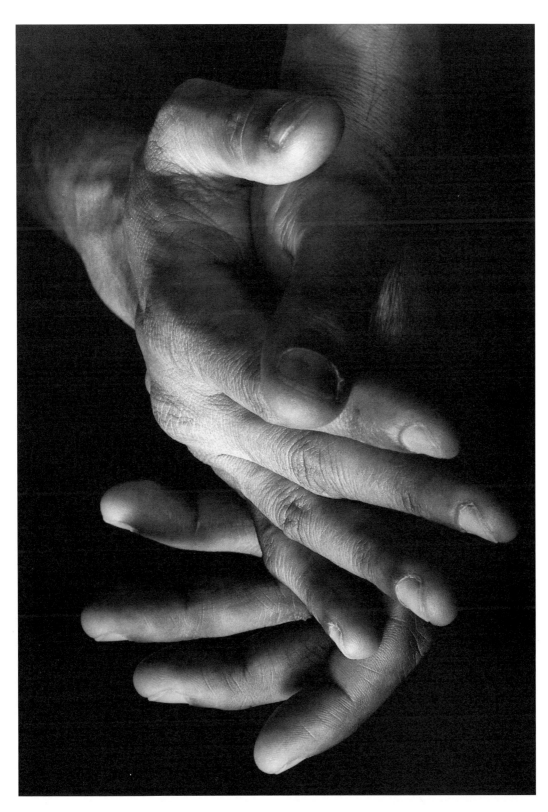

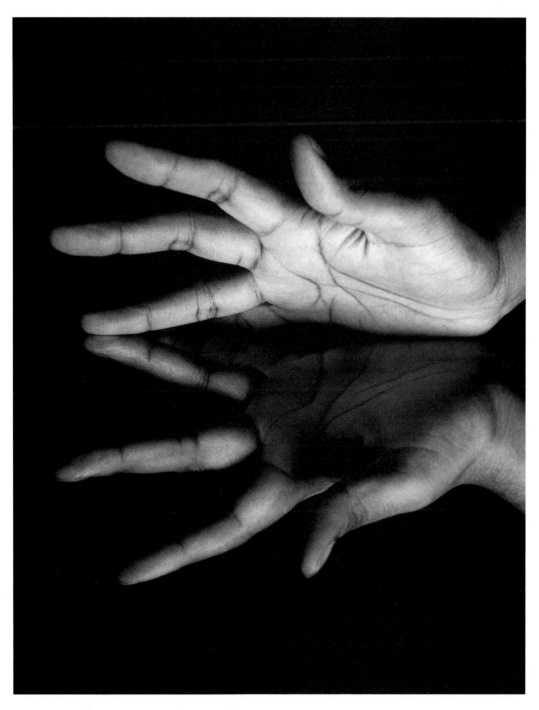

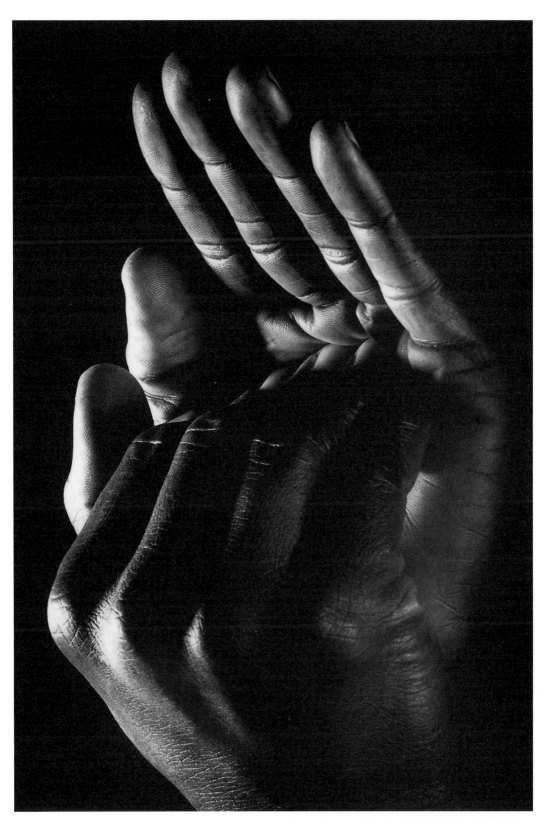

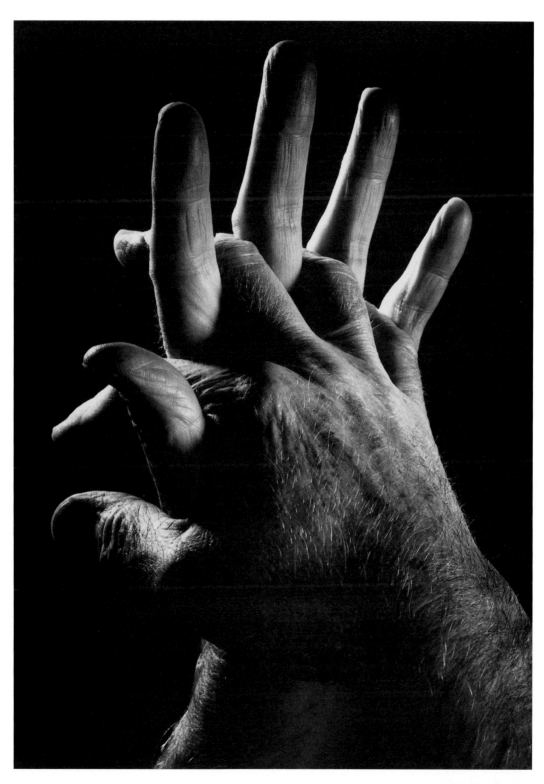

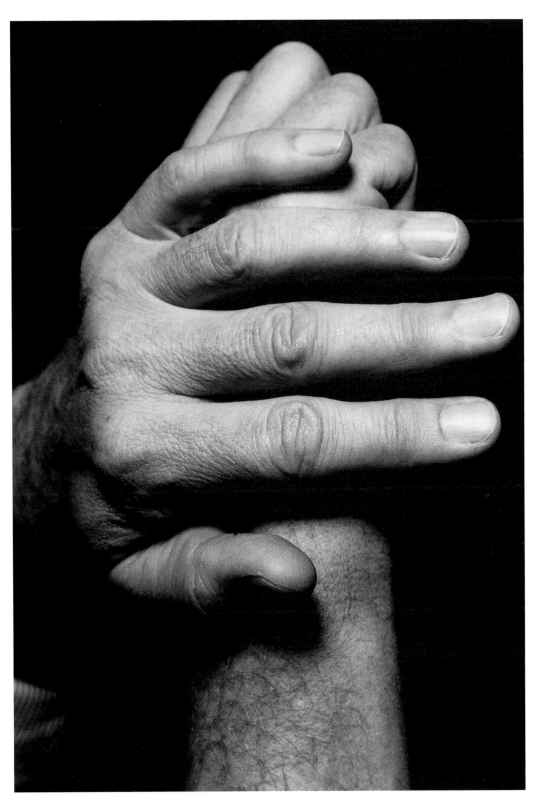

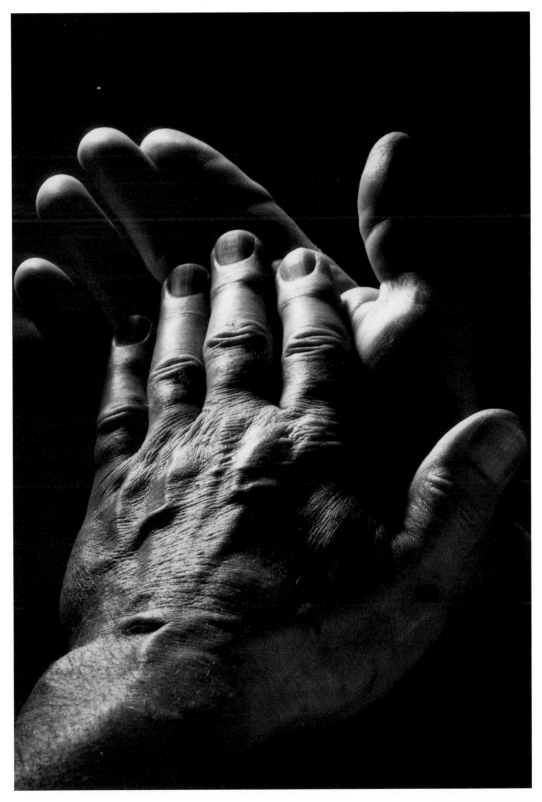

STEIN, BENNETT   *153*

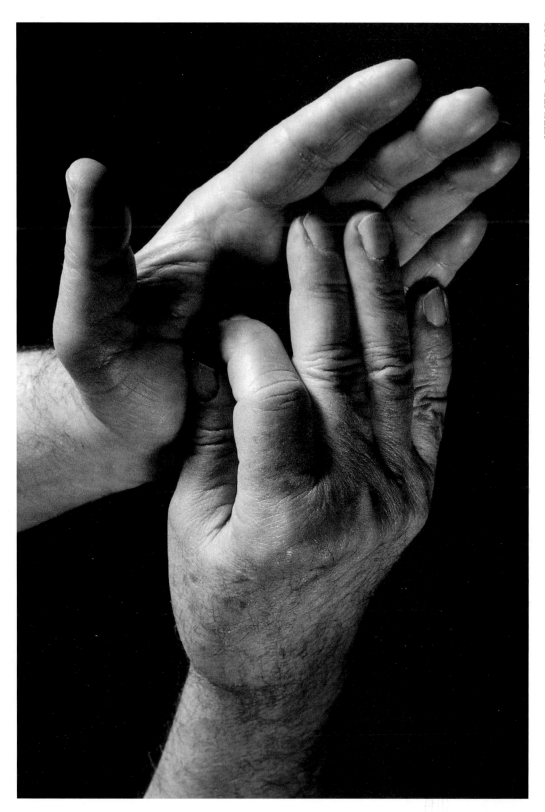

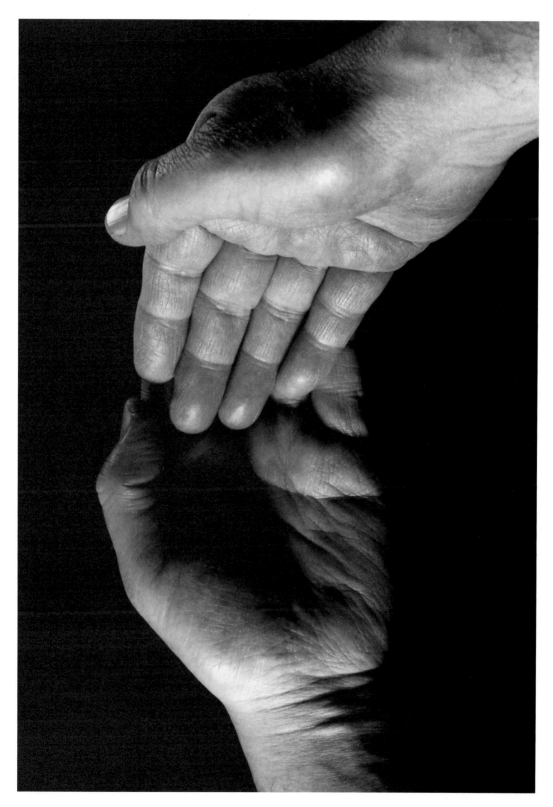

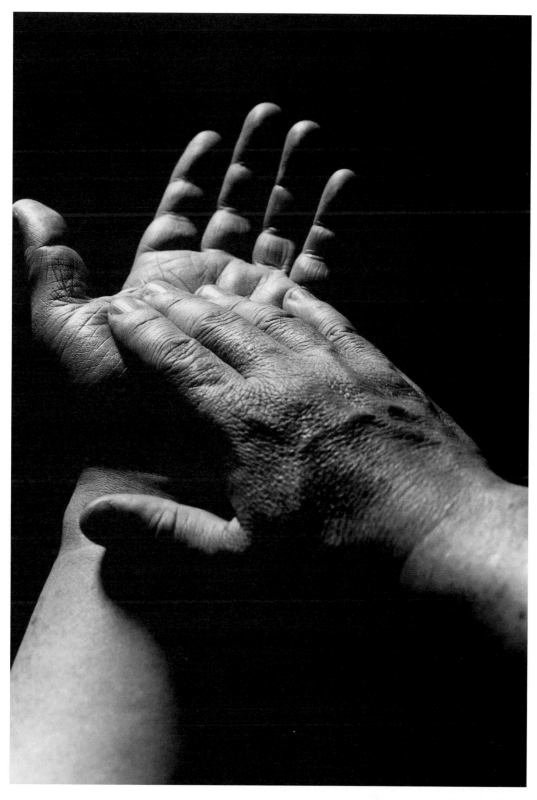

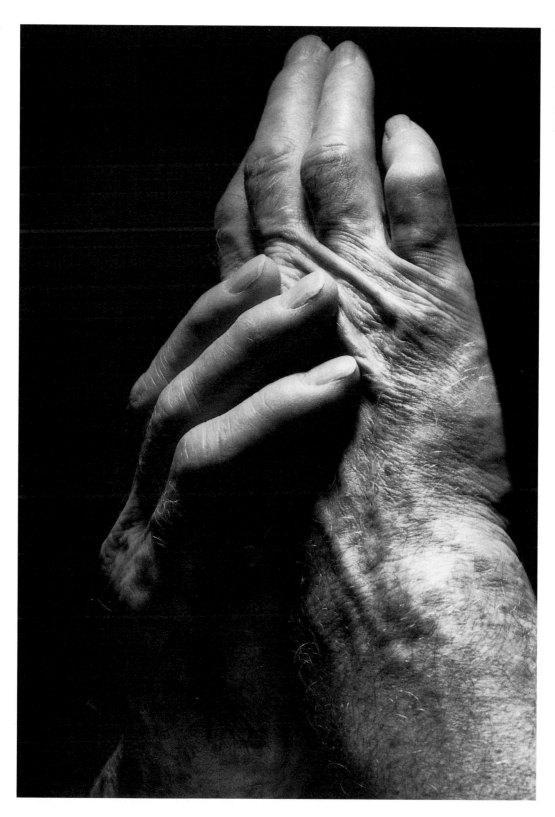

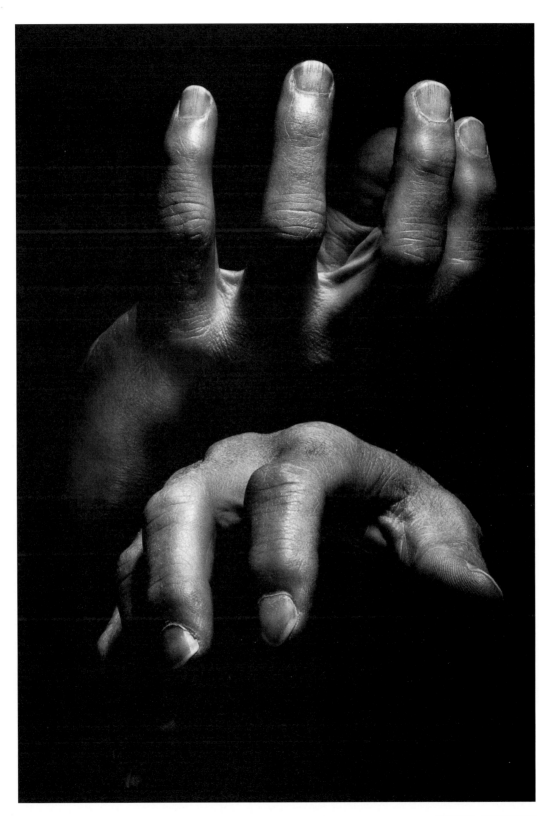

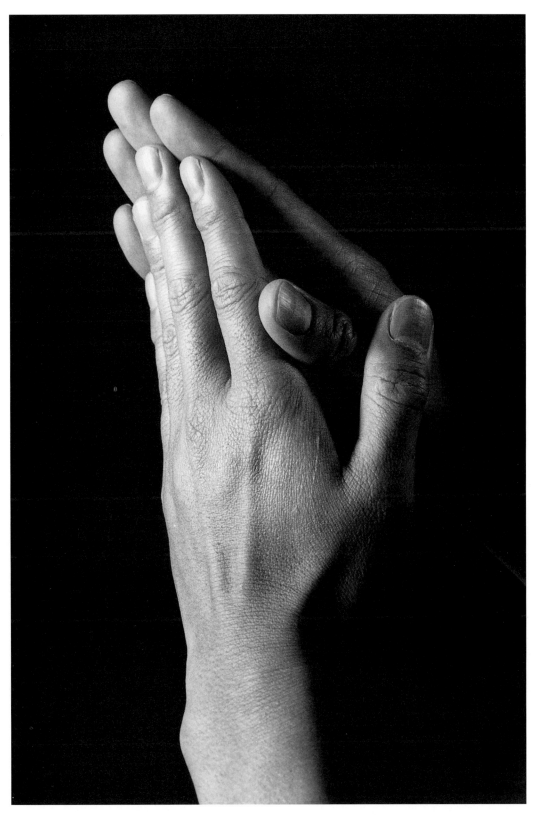

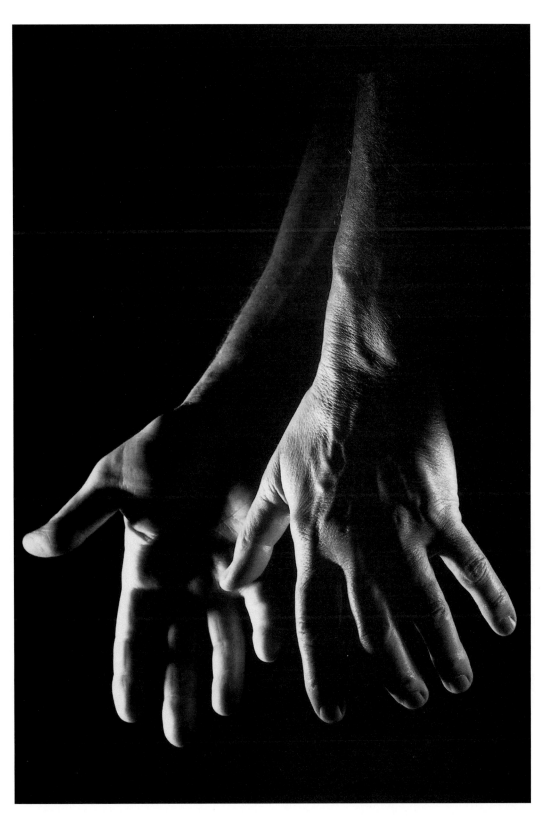

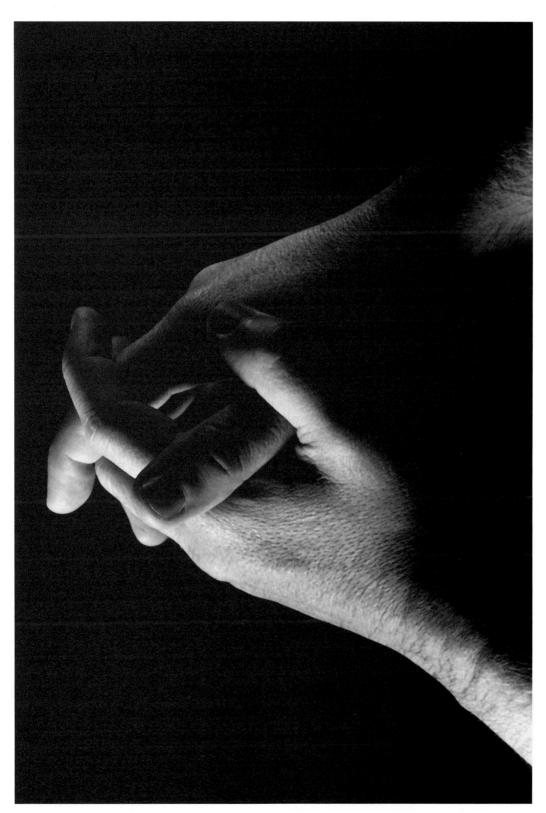

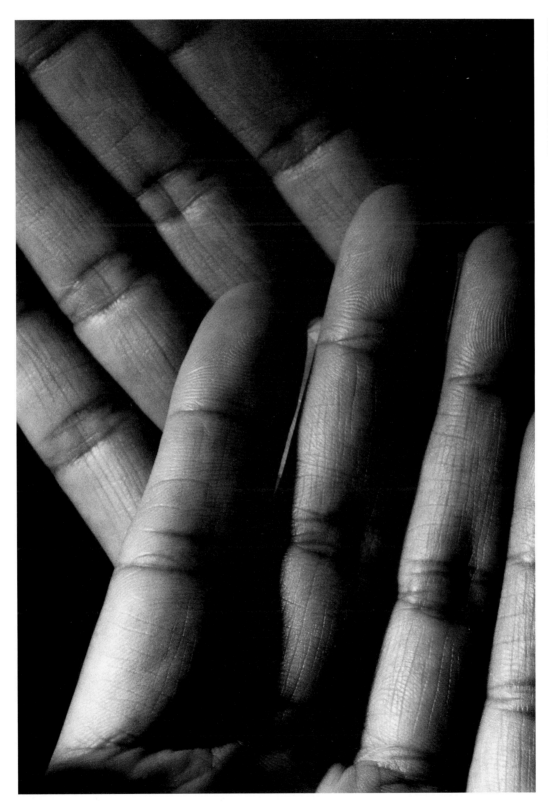

VAN LOVEREN, HARRY

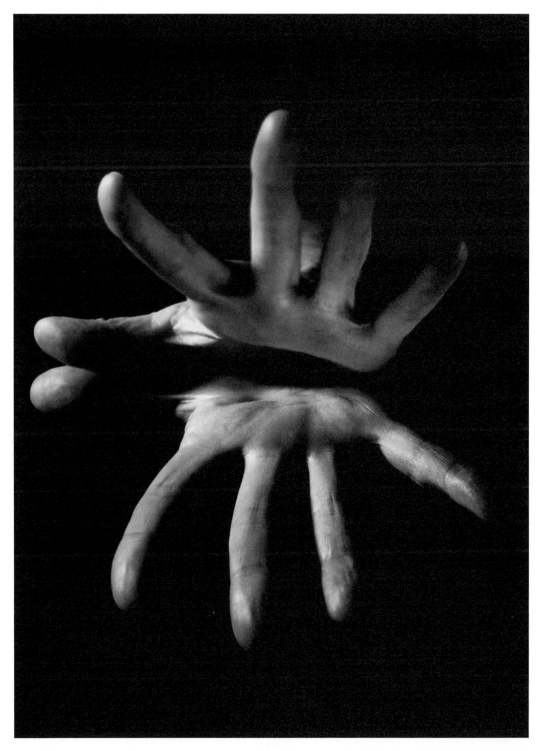

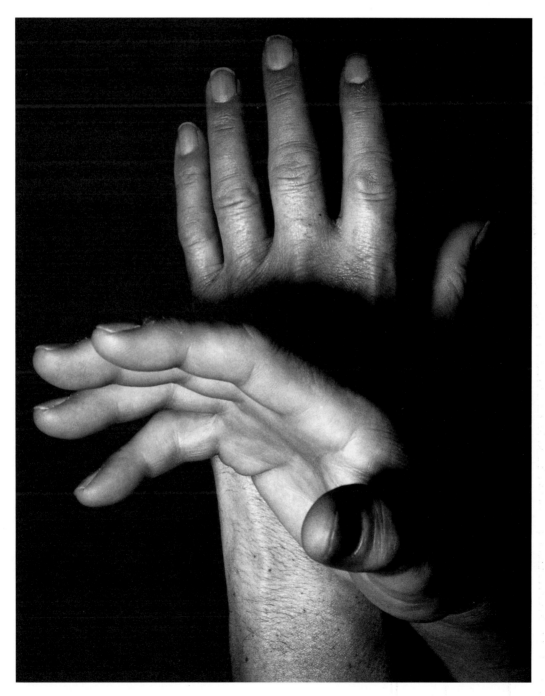

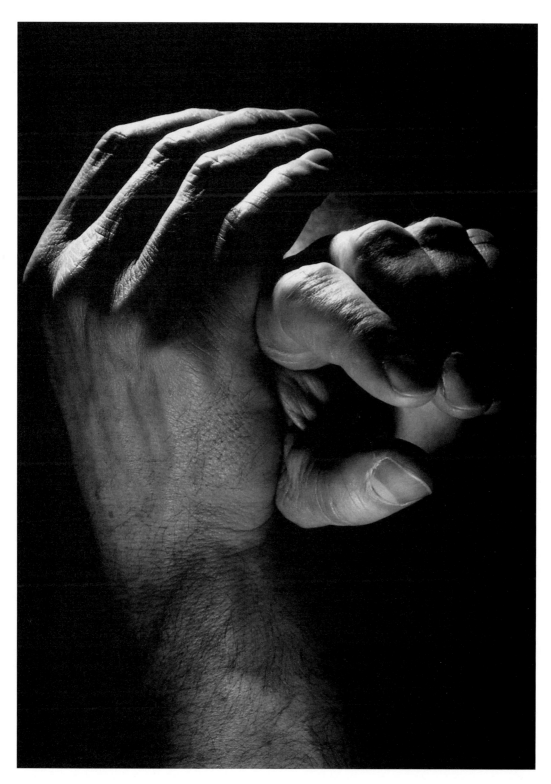

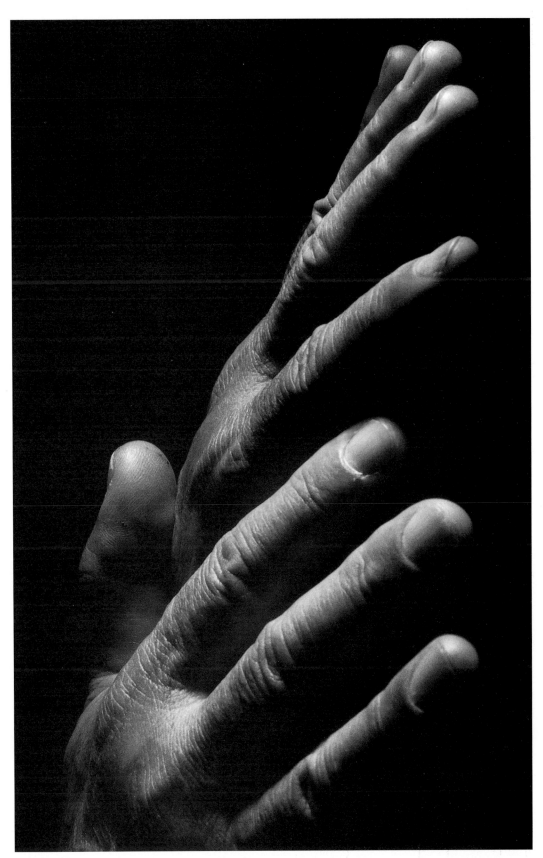

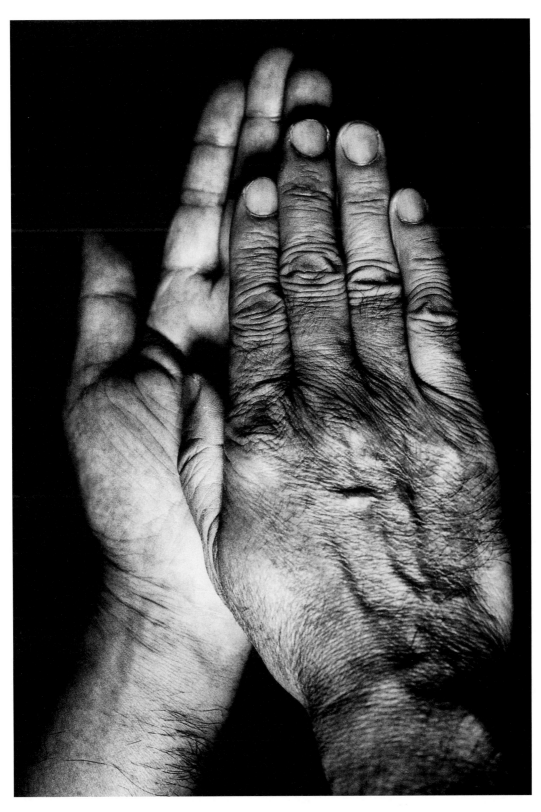

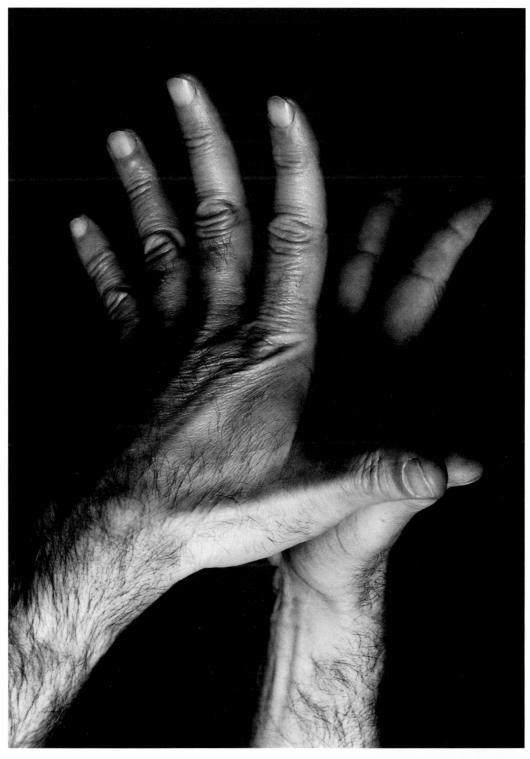

PORTRAIT INDEX

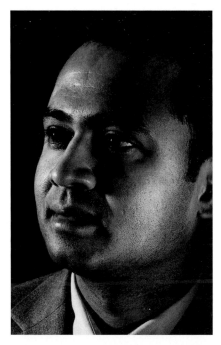

ABDULRAUF, SALEEM
St. Louis, Missouri, US
p. 3

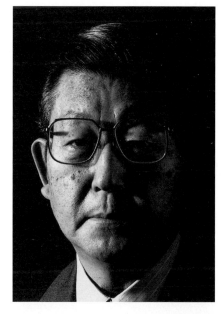

ABE, HIROSHI
Sapporo, Japan
p. 5

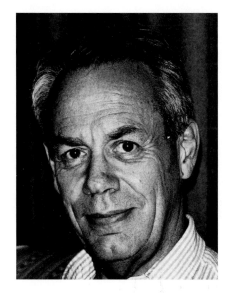

ADAMS, CHRISTOPHER
Oxford, England
p. 7

187

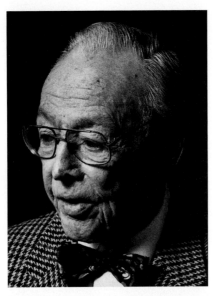

ALEXANDER, EBEN, JR.
Winston-Salem, North Carolina, US
p. 9

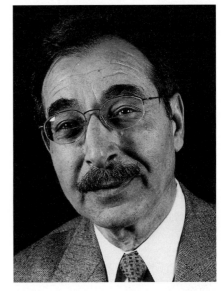

AL-MEFTY, OSSAMA
Little Rock, Arkansas, US
p. 11

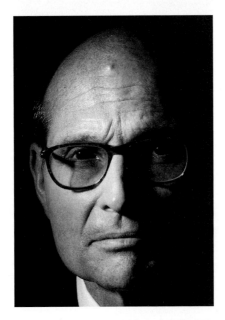

APUZZO, MICHAEL
Los Angeles, California, US
p. 13

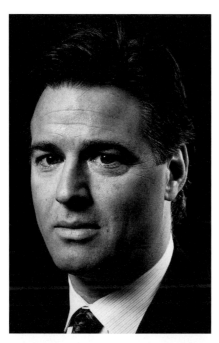

BARROW, DANIEL
Atlanta, Georgia, US
p. 15

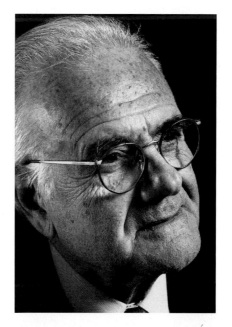

BASSO, ARMANDO
Buenos Aires, Argentina
p. 17

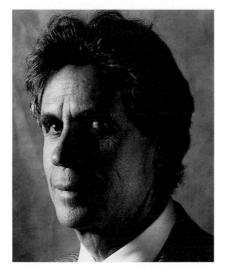

BECKER, DONALD
Los Angeles, California, US
p. 19

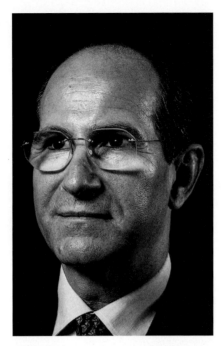

BENABID, ALIM-LOUIS
Grenoble, France
p. 21

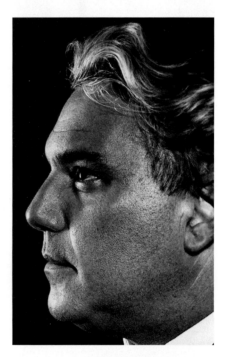

BERGER, MITCHEL
San Francisco, California, US
p. 23

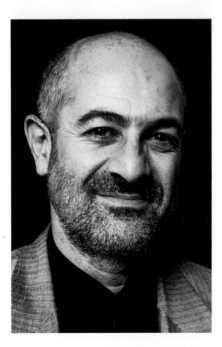

BERNSTEIN, MARK
Toronto, Ontario, Canada
p. 25

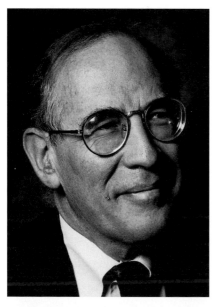

BLACK, PETER
Boston, Massachusetts, US
p. 27

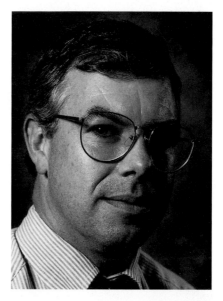

BOOP, FREDERICK
Memphis, Tennessee, US
p. 29

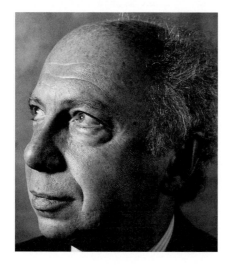

BROTCHI, JACQUES
Brussels, Belgium
p.31

191

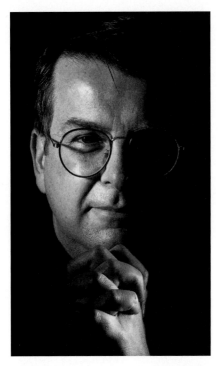

BUCHOLZ, RICHARD
St. Louis, Missouri, US
p. 33

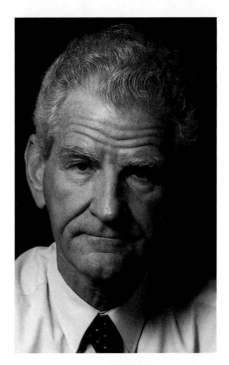

CHOUX, MAURICE
Marseilles, France
p. 35

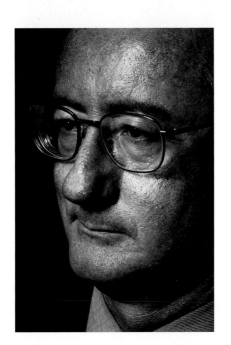

COLOHAN, AUSTIN
Loma Linda, California, US
p. 37

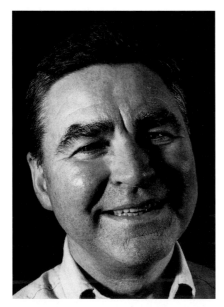

CROCKARD, ALAN
London, England
p. 39

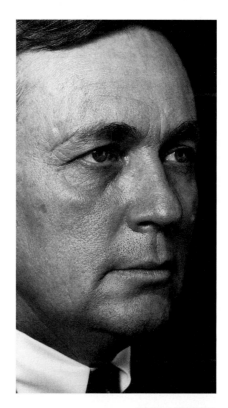

DAY, ARTHUR
Gainesville, Florida, US
p. 41

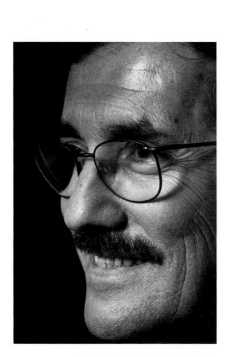

DE OLIVEIRA, EVANDRO
Sao Paulo, Brazil
p. 43

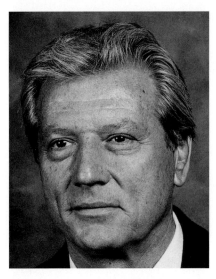

DOLENC, VINKO
Charlottesville, Virginia, US
p. 45

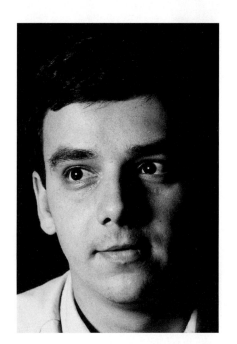

DOSOUTO, ANTONIO
Rio De Janeiro, Brazil
p. 47

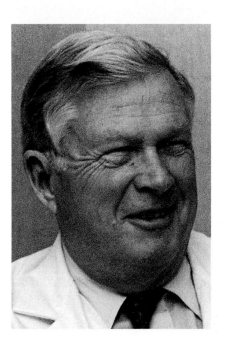

DRAKE, CHARLES
London, Ontario, Canada
p. 49

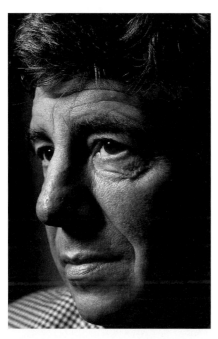

FAHLBUSCH, RUDOLPH
Erlangen, Germany
p. 51

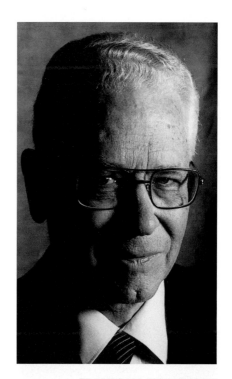

FLANIGAN, STEVENSON
Harrison, Arkansas, US
p. 53

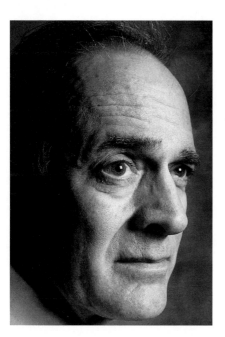

FOX, JOHN
Little Rock, Arkansas, US
p. 55

195

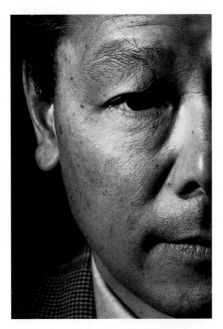

FUKUSHIMA, TAKANORI
Raleigh, North Carolina, US
p. 57

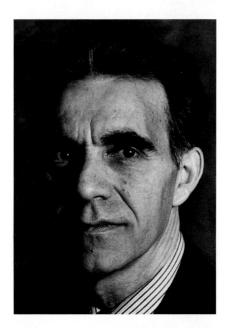

GENTILI, FRED
Toronto, Ontario, Canada
p. 59

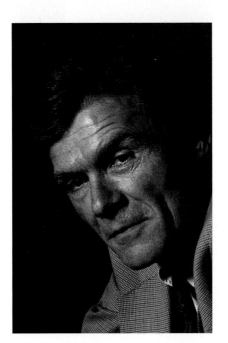

GEORGE, BERNARD
Paris, France
p. 61

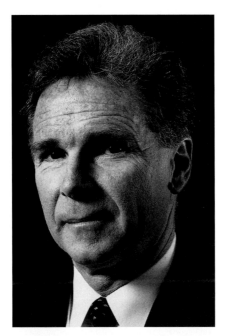

GIANNOTTA, STEVEN
Los Angeles, California, US
p. 63

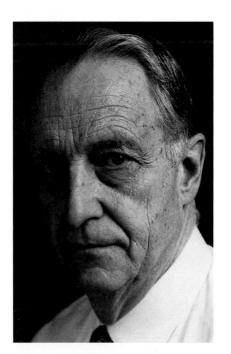

GIRVIN, JOHN
London, Ontario, Canada
p. 65

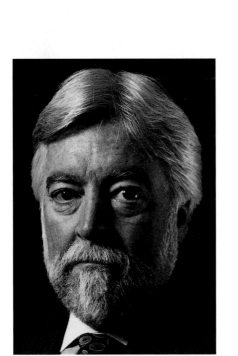

GOODRICH, JAMES
Bronx, New York, US
p. 67

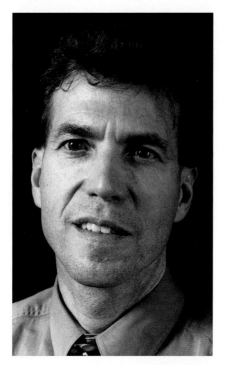

GOPLEN, GARY
Kelowna, British Columbia, Canada
p. 69

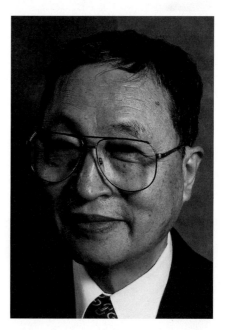

HAKUBA, AKIRA
Osaka, Japan
p. 71

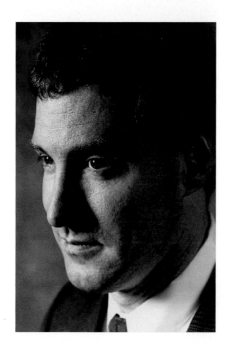

HARRISON, MICHAEL
Vancouver, Washington, US
p. 73

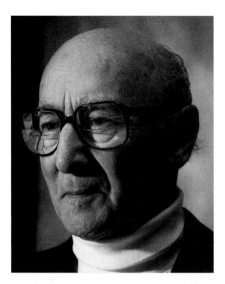

HEIFETZ, MILTON
Beverly Hills, California, US
p. 75

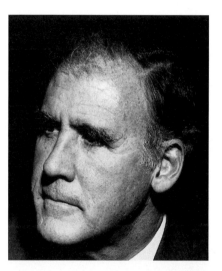

HEROS, ROBERTO
Miami, Florida, US
p. 77

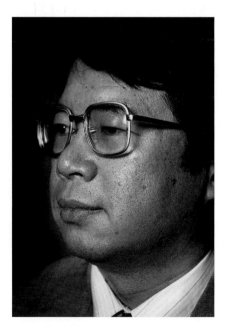

HONGO, KAZUHIRO
Matsumoto, Japan
p. 79

199

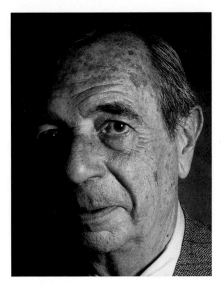

ISAMAT, FABIAN
Barcelona, Spain
p. 81

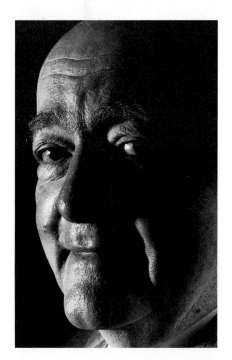

JANE, JOHN
Charlottesville, Virginia, US
p. 83

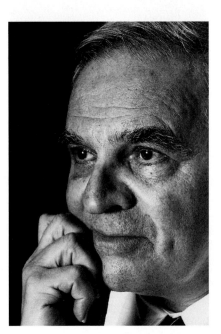

JANNETTA, PETER
Pittsburgh, Pennsylvania, US
p. 85

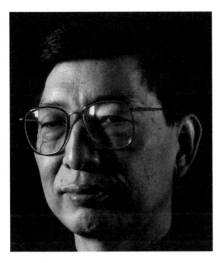

JHO, HAE-DONG
Pittsburgh, Pennsylvania, US
p. 87

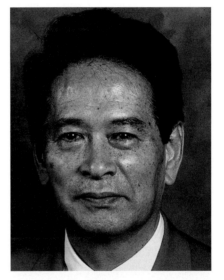

KANNO, TETSUO
Aichi, Japan
p. 89

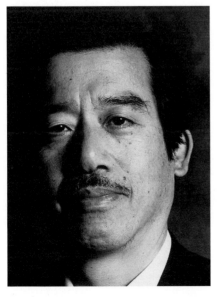

KAWASE, TAKESHI
Tokyo, Japan
p. 91

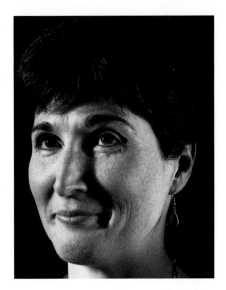

KISS, ZELMA
Calgary, Alberta, Canada
p. 93

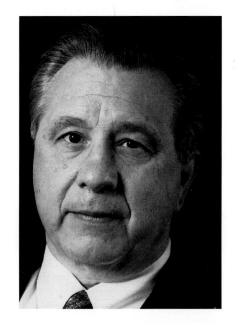

KLINE, DAVID
New Orleans, Louisiana, US
p. 95

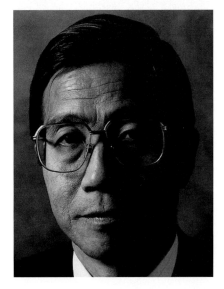

KOBAYASHI, SHIGEAKI
Matsumoto, Japan
p. 97

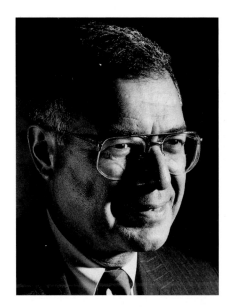

LAWS, EDWARD
Charlottesville, Virginia, US
p. 99

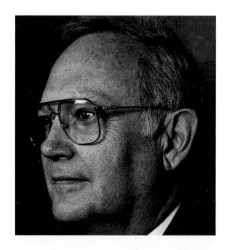

LONG, DONLIN
Baltimore, Maryland, US
p. 101

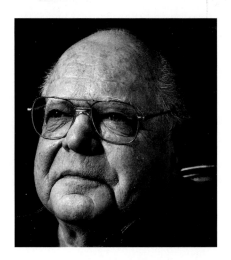

LOUGHEED, WILLIAM
Barrie, Ontario, Canada
p. 103

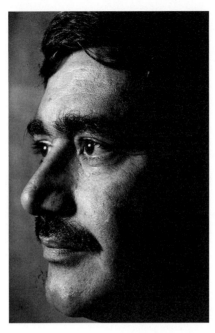

MALIK, AYAZ
Garland, Texas, US
p. 105

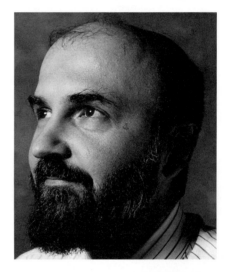

MALIK, JACEK
Salisbury, Maryland, US
p. 107

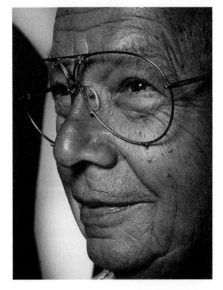

MALIS, LEONARD
New York, New York, US
p. 109

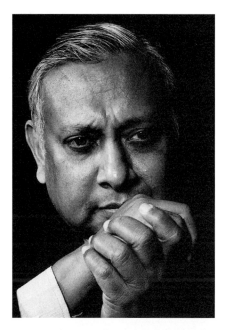

MENEZES, ARNOLD
Iowa City, Iowa, US
p. 111

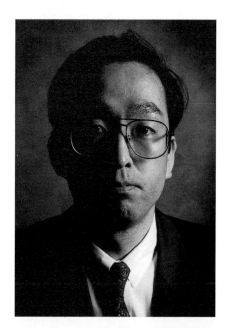

NAKASE, HIROYUKI
Japan
p. 113

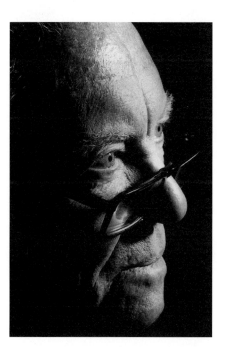

NUGENT, ROBERT
Morgantown, West Virginia, US
p. 115

205

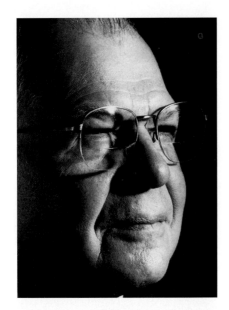

OJEMANN, ROBERT
Boston, Massachusetts, US
p. 117

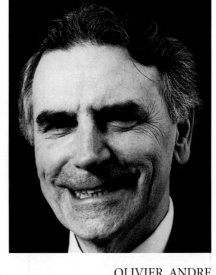

OLIVIER, ANDRE
Montreal, Quebec, Canada
p. 119

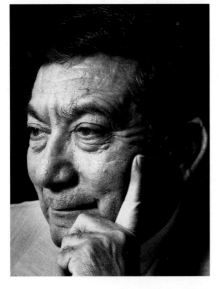

OMMAYA, AYUB
Bethesda, Maryland, US
p. 121

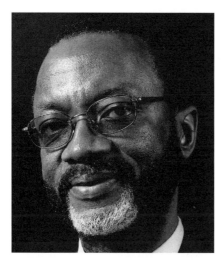

ORDIA, JOE
Boston, Massachusetts, US
p. 123

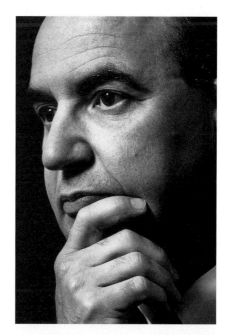

ORO, JOHN
Columbia, Missouri, US
p. 125

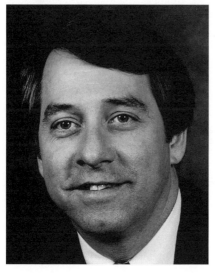

PAIT, T. GLENN
Little Rock, Arkansas, US
p. 127

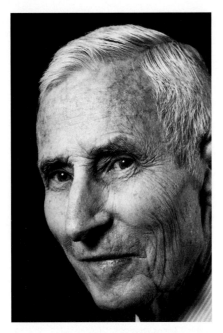

PARKINSON, DWIGHT
Winnipeg, Manitoba, Canada
p. 129

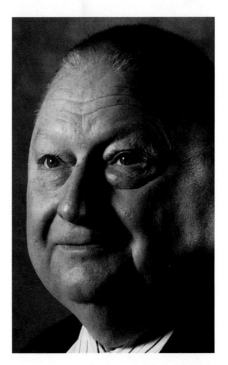

REICHMAN, HOWARD
Provo, Utah, US
p. 131

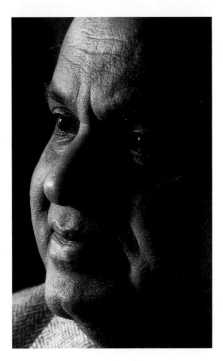

RENGACHARY, SETTI
Detroit, Michigan, US
p. 133

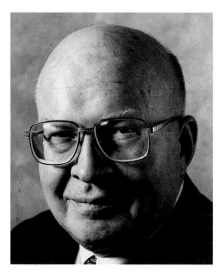

RHOTON, ALBERT
Gainseville, Florida, US
p. 135

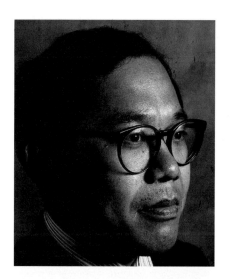

SAKATA, KATSUMI
Okinawa, Japan
p. 137

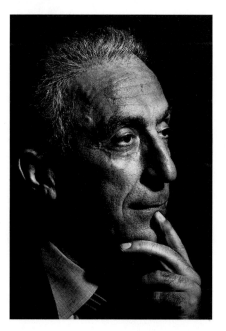

SAMII, MADJID
Hanover, Germany
p. 139

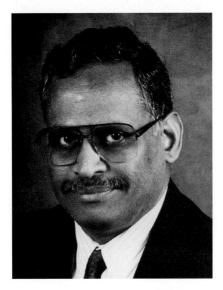

SEKHAR, LALIGAM
Fairfax, Virginia, US
p. 141

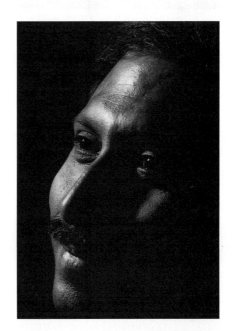

SEN, CHANDRANATH
New York, New York, US
p. 143

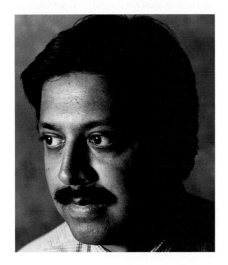

SIDDIQI, JAVED
Colton, California, US
p. 145

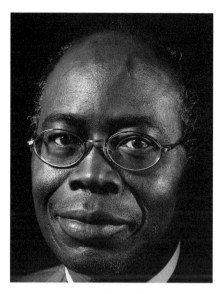

SMART-ABBEY, VICTOR
Long Beach, California, US
p. 147

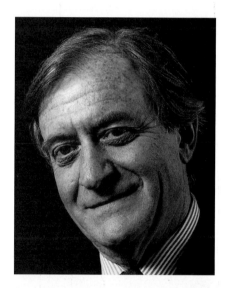

SMYTH, HARLEY
Toronto, Ontario, Canada
p. 149

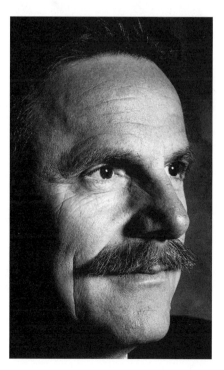

SPETZLER, ROBERT
Phoenix, Arizona, US
p. 151

211

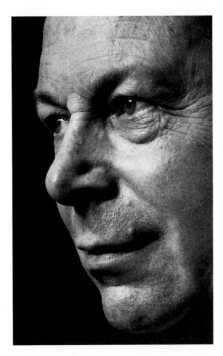

STEIN, BENNETT
New York, New York, US
p. 153

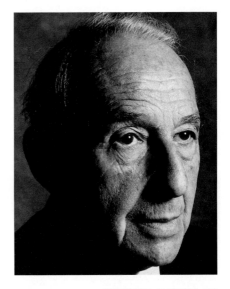

STEINER, LADISLAU
Charlottesville, Florida, US
p. 155

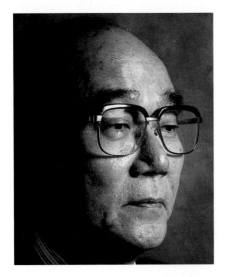

TAKAKURA, KINTOMO
Tokyo, Japan

212   *p. 157*

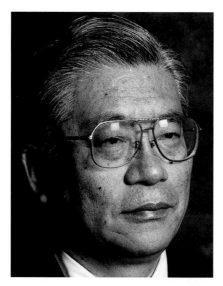

TAMAKI, NORIHIKO
Kobe, Japan
p. 159

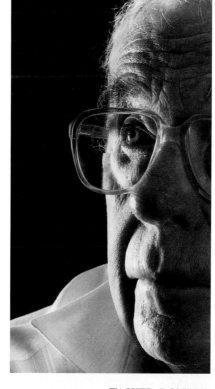

TASKER, RONALD
Toronto, Ontario, Canada
p. 161

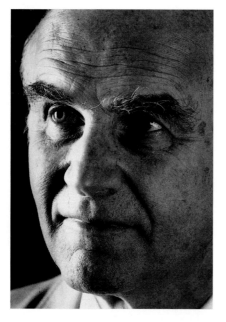

TATOR, CHARLES
Toronto, Ontario, Canada
p. 163

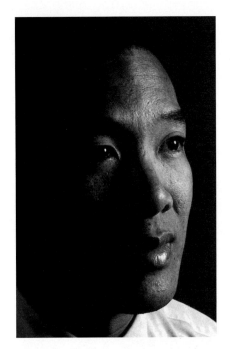

TEO, CHARLES
Sydney, Australia
p. 165

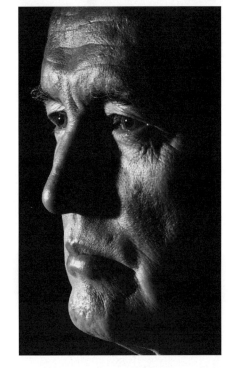

TEW, JOHN, JR.
Cincinnati, Ohio, US
p. 167

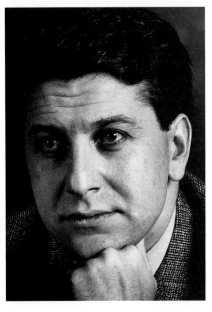

TURE, UGUR
Istanbul, Turkey
p. 169

214

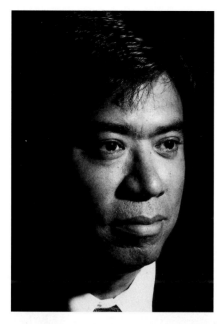

VAN LOVEREN, HARRY
Cincinnati, Ohio, US
p. 171

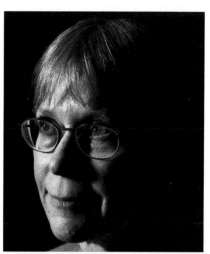

WALTERS, BEVERLY
Providence, Rhode Island, US
p. 173

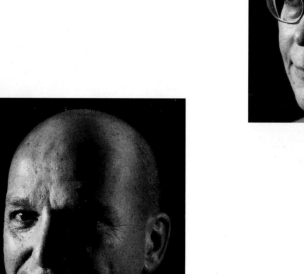

WEISS, MARTIN
Los Angeles, California, US
p. 175

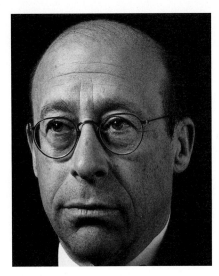

WINN, RICHARD
Seattle, Washington, US
p. 177

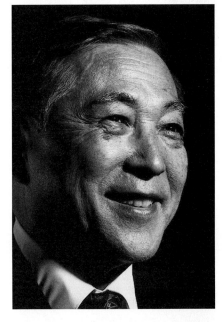

YAMADA, SHOKEI
Loma Linda, California, US
p. 179

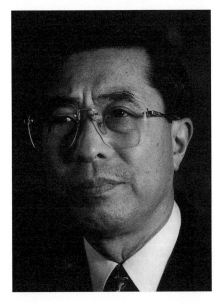

YAMAMOTO, ISAO
Yokohama, Japan
p. 181

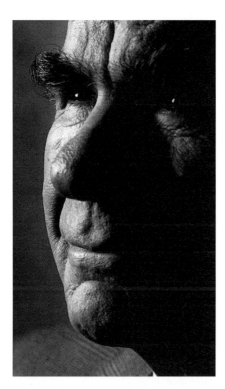

YASARGIL, GAZI
Little Rock, Arkansas, US
p. 183